TOPICS IN Clinical Nursing

Death and Dying

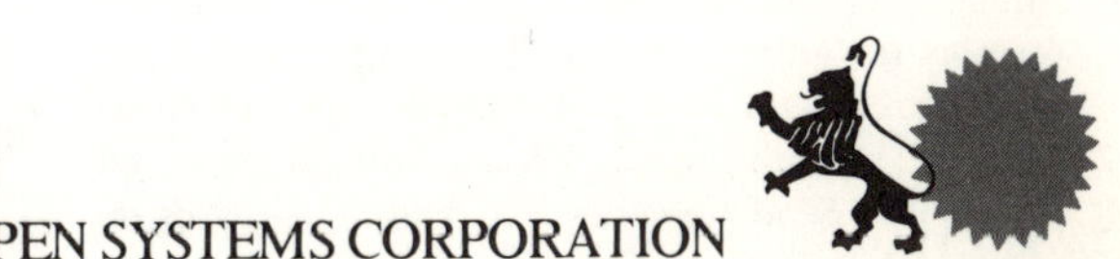

ASPEN SYSTEMS CORPORATION

TOPICS IN
Clinical Nursing

An Aspen Publication®

Publisher: Theodore Caris
Editor-in-Chief: John R. Marozsan
Editorial Director: N. Darlene Como
Managing Editor: Margot S. Raphael
Senior Editor: Susan S. Rosenberg

Editorial Assistant: Lorraine B. Davis
Production Manager: Paul R. Carlin
Manager Fulfillment Operations:
Ernest V. Manzella, Jr.

TOPICS IN CLINICAL NURSING (USPS 474-850) is published quarterly for $29.00 per year by Aspen Systems Corporation, 16792 Oakmont Avenue Gaithersburg, Maryland 20877. Second-class postage paid at Gaithersburg, Maryland, and additional mailing offices. POSTMASTER: Send address changes to Aspen Systems Corporation, 16792 Oakmont Avenue, Gaithersburg, MD 20877.

Subscription rates: $29.00 per year in the United States and Canada (four issues), payable in advance. Subscribers may specify any issue to begin the subscription. **Subscribers in United Kingdom, Europe, Middle East and Africa:** Aspen Systems Corporation, 3 Henrietta Street, London WC2E 8LU, ENGLAND. Delivered subscription prices available on request. **Subscribers in Japan:** Address subscription inquiries to Maruzen Company, Ltd., P.O. Box 5050, Tokyo International, 100-31, JAPAN.

Editorial correspondence, letters to the editor, and manuscript submissions should be addressed to: Editorial Director, TCN, Aspen Systems Corporation, 1600 Research Boulevard, Rockville, Maryland 20850.

Business correspondence (subscription inquiries, subscription orders, change of address, etc.) should be addressed to Fulfillment Operations, Aspen Systems Corporation, 16792 Oakmont Avenue, Gaithersburg, MD 20877.

Notices for change of address, including the subscriber's old and new address, should be sent to Fulfillment Operations, Aspen Systems Corporation, 16792 Oakmont Avenue, Gaithersburg, MD 20877, six weeks in advance of effective date.

Single copies: $12.00 each; enclose payment with order. **Single issue for educational use** (minimum order of five copies): $8.95. **Multiple copies for educational and training programs:** Inquiries from bona fide educational programs concerning terms of sale will be answered promptly. Send inquiries to Fulfillment Operations, Aspen Systems Corporation, 16792 Oakmont Avenue, Gaithersburg, MD 20877.

Advertising: Journal Advertising Sales Department 4A, Aspen Systems Corporation, 1600 Research Boulevard, Rockville, MD 20850. Telephone: (301) 251-5000.

Microform: This publication is available in microform from University Microfilms International, 300 North Zeeb Road, Dept. P.R., Ann Arbor, MI 48106. Article reprints are also available from University Microfilms International, Article Reprint Services, at the same address.

Issue: Vol. 3, No. 3 ISBN: 0-89443-210-9
ISSN: 0164-0534
Printed in the United States of America.

Contents

Death and Dying

Editorial board

Jane Bragdon Hanron, BSN, MEd
Boston College School of Nursing
Department of Continuing Education
Chestnut Hill, Massachusetts

Sandra H. Hanson, BSN, MEd
Assistant Professor
Department of Pediatric Nursing
College of Health Sciences
School of Nursing
University of Kansas
Kansas City, Kansas

Jeanette Lancaster, RN, PhD
Professor and Chairman
MSN Degree Program
School of Nursing
University of Alabama
Birmingham, Alabama

Anthony Mascia, RN, MSN
Clinical Nurse Specialist, Pediatrics
Maternal-Child Health Consultant
Visiting Nurse Association of Hartford, Inc.
Hartford, Connecticut

Mary A. McClelland, RN, MA
Director of Nursing Services
Parma Community General Hospital
Parma, Ohio

Andrea Mengel, RN, MSN
Assistant Professor of Nursing
Community College of Philadelphia
Philadelphia, Pennsylvania

M. Janice Nelson, RN, EdD
Associate Administrator for Nursing
State University Hospital
Upstate Medical Center
Syracuse, New York

Annalee R. Oakes, RN, MA, CCRN
Associate Professor of Nursing
Clinical Instructor of Emergency-Critical
   Care Nursing
Seattle Pacific University
Seattle, Washington

Teresa Ann Peduzzi, RN, MSN
Chairperson
Department of Nursing
Erie Institute for Nursing
Villa Maria College
Erie, Pennsylvania

Gretchen Randolph, RN, PhD
Consultant, Private Practice
Randolph-Price and Associates
Portland, Oregon

William R. Stayton, MDiv, ThD
Assistant Professor of Psychiatry and
   Human Behavior
Department of Psychiatry
Thomas Jefferson University Medical College
Philadelphia, Pennsylvania

Alice M. Stein, RN, MA
Director of Continuing Nursing Education
The Medical College of Pennsylvania
Philadelphia, Pennsylvania

Theresa M. Valiga, RN, EdM
Assistant Professor of Nursing
Director, Undergraduate Program
College of Nursing
Seton Hall University
South Orange, New Jersey

Zane M. Robinson Wolf, RN, MSN
Assistant Professor
La Salle College Nursing Program
Philadelphia, Pennsylvania

Nancy Fugate Woods, RN, PhD
Associate Professor
School of Nursing
University of Washington
Seattle, Washington

From the editors

This issue on death and dying is a joyful one. It represents how a holistic perspective enriches the practice of nursing. Presented here is a collection of articles in which death is considered a natural part of living rather than a dread to be denied and avoided at all cost.

Care of the dying is a major source of stress for health care professionals. It reminds us of our own inevitable end. Caring for the dying in acute care settings, where the value of curing is so much higher than the value of caring, is even more difficult. The acute care setting often traps nurses into sacrificing support measures for client and family to treatment regimes that prolong and even try to standardize the dying process.

The most important message of this issue is that ways of dying are as unique as individuals themselves. Some people fight, some slip off quietly in sleep. Some families are stoic, others are strident in their grief, and others embed the mourning process in ritual.

There will never be a clinically standardized way of dying. The best way to improve our care of the dying is to attempt to understand this human process in all its dimensions. This issue will help those who seek to understand more.

—Doris C. Sutterley, RN, MSN
—Gloria F. Donnelly, RN, MSN
Editors

Letters to the editor

All letters to the editor should be addressed to: Editor, TCN, Aspen Systems Corporation, 1600 Research Boulevard, Rockville, MD 20850. Unless otherwise noted, we assume that letters addressed to the editor are intended for publication with your name and affiliation. As many letters as possible will be published. When space is limited and we cannot publish all letters received, we will select letters reflecting the range of opinions and ideas received. If a letter merits a response from a TCN author, we will obtain a reply and publish both letters.

Foreword

Few occurrences in this world have greater emotional impact on the living than the final event of death. The process of dying begins when one is born and continues at various rates according to the uniqueness of the organism and the conditions of the environment. Usually death is associated with sadness and tears and almost never celebrated with joy. Death may be anticipated or unexpected, but all living things eventually die.

Nurses, because of the nature of their practice environments and the physical and emotional qualities of patient care, are situationally positioned to encounter high levels of contact with the process of death and dying. They are vulnerable, more than most other professionals, to the "sting of death."

The articles included in this issue are intended to stimulate discussion and reflection on selected concepts of death and dying. The authors have amassed a diversity of information to expand the nurse's scope of working knowledge, explore strategies and methods for nursing intervention, and encourage a sensitivity to consider one's own orientation to this life process. An extensive overview of societal/cultural views of death and dying creates a rich background from which nurses can glean insights into the individuality and uniquenesses of the death experience. Various peoples from Western cultures as well as lesser known anthropologic groups are presented in dialogue and prose. The social organization of care for the dying, working with dying patients in acute illness frameworks, community impact with death loss of infants and medico-legal considerations are issues of care delivery addressed.

An article about a person's need of faith at the time of death, written by a philosopher-theologian, helps to direct nursing toward holistic care in which patients maintain hope to the end of life. Medico-legal considerations and the quality of life challenge the reader to make decisions about clinical dilemmas surrounding when and how life will be terminated.

Nurses are continually expanding into new and uncharted areas of practice. The discussion of near-death phenomena and critical care nursing practice offers a pioneering view of another dimension still to be studied but very much a part of clinical scenes today.

Few journals recognize the sensitive input of families who, sharing their last days with a loved one, encourage the help and appreciation of care givers ministering to the dying. This issue presents a moving account of such a family—the final days and the responses of the dying person to their love and support.

The concluding article focuses on the process of death education throughout the professional development of nurses. Traditionally, nursing education taught suppression of any discussion of feelings and personal involvement with the dying patient. Nurses were directed to prepare the body for the hospital morgue and not discuss any details with the family while attempting to gain permission for an autopsy as quickly as possible. Today, knowledge and clinical involvement with patients who are in the process of dying and their families throughout the pre- and post-death period are crucial to developing a holistic nursing care practice.

Living experiences, culture, religion, theory concepts and clinical practice methods are presented here. The authors recognize that in the American society and health care system, the nurse is in the awesome and strategic position of receiving an overwhelming exposure to death. Nurses, capable and willing to learn new ways of helping the patient, are still the most sophisticated advocates for providing a better quality of life for patients and their families as they live the process of dying. This issue is dedicated to them . . . care givers bridging the transition from this life into death.

—Annalee Oakes, RN, MA, CCRN
—Clarann Weinert, SC, RN, MA, PhC
  Issue Editors

Ms. Oakes teaches Emergency Critical Care Nursing at Seattle Pacific University, Seattle, Washington. She was a national treasurer and board member for the American Association of Critical Care Nurses, and is a member of the American Heart Association and an Affiliate Faculty of Advanced Cardiac Life Support, American Heart Association.

Sister Clarann Weinert is a doctoral candidate in the department of Sociology at the University of Washington in Seattle, Washington.

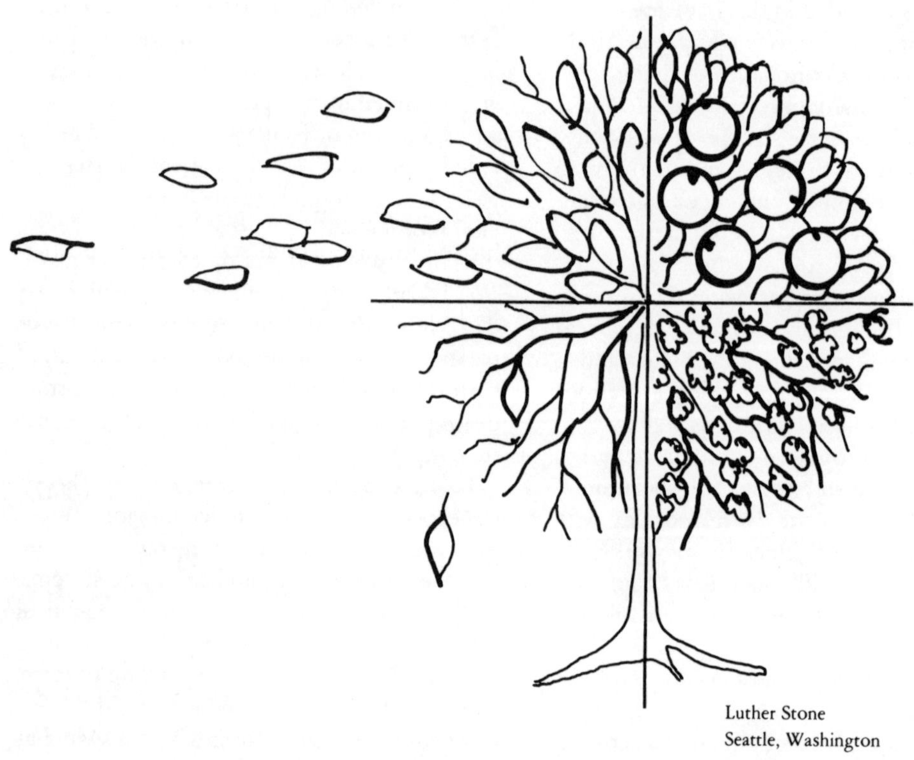

Luther Stone
Seattle, Washington

Societal/cultural views regarding death and dying

H. Miriam Ross, RN, MS, MA, PhC
Graduate Student
Department of Anthropology
University of Washington
Seattle, Washington

AT DUSK, four weary men carefully set down the litter in the hospital courtyard. For six hours they had walked over hilly terrain carrying a semiconscious young woman who had been in labor for three days. Now the woman was convulsing; there was no fetal heartbeat. Throughout the night hospital staff worked desperately to save the woman's life. At dawn she died. Amid the keening wails of distraught relatives, the exhausted medical staff started home to get some rest. The family looked at the body, then ran after the surgeon.

"You didn't take the baby out of the mother!"

"Of course not. Why should I?"

"You have to do that. We can't bury the mother with the baby still inside her."

The surgeon and nurse-midwife, both Americans, were astonished and appalled.

"But it's the way it has to be done. It's the law! We won't take the body unless you take out the baby."

The surgeon contacted an attorney. The

0164-0534/81/0033-0001$2.00
© 1981 Aspen Systems Corporation

attorney said, "It's not legally required, but it's their custom."

The family insisted; the surgeon refused. An impasse. Finally, after much negotiation, the relatives called an indigenous doctor who removed the fetus so that they could bury the infant separately from its mother.

Although this incident took place on a Caribbean island, it highlights the conflicts that can arise when care seekers and care givers hold different cultural assumptions. That situation often occurs in the United States today. No longer a "melting pot," the country is now a "micro-world reflecting the cultural diversity of the entire larger world."[1] To accommodate such diversity, medical professionals need to employ a cross-cultural perspective. From that vantage point, care givers can break free of reliance solely upon their own meager slice of reason and experience.

The term *culture* is used in many different ways.[2] One useful definition of culture is "an integrated system of learned patterns of behavior, ideas, and products characteristic of a society."[3]

Culture influences death concerns in a myriad of ways:

- It affects the assessment of comfort needs of the dying and the kind of care provided.
- It influences selection, perception and evaluation of health care givers and their methods.
- It shapes beliefs about causes of death.
- It determines the disposition of the body and funeral and burial rituals.
- It patterns grief responses and bereavement roles.

In fact, Kalish claims that it is "impossible to exaggerate the role of culture" in death and dying.[4] Furthermore, behaviors surrounding death and bereavement are among cultural features that are the "most conservative and most resistant to change."[5]

The fact of death is singular; the ways of death are multiform. Like the aged in primitive society, an individual may "deny death as a natural necessity, resist it as a curse, submit to it as the hand of fate, embrace it as a golden opportunity, or even demand it as a right."[6] The dying may be ignored, isolated, abandoned, neglected, feared, despised or eliminated; or they may be loved, protected, cherished and succored until the moment of expiration. Whatever the way of death, culture plays a prominent role in the decisions and behaviors of the persons involved.

ACCOUNTS OF DEATH IN OTHER CULTURES

Medical professionals have described some of the ways in which people in other cultures cope with death. Some of these mechanisms appear detrimental to well-being; others might be helpful in meeting problems within western culture. Accounts range from subterfuges used in Iran to conceal from the patient any suspicion of impending death to ways by which acceptance of death is built into the entire life span of Aymara Indians in Bolivia.[7,8] The Xhosa of South Africa conceive of death as a journey: "Preparation is all-important, as for any journey; to them there appears no reason to hang on to the last few weeks of life, provided they are ready for the journey."[9]

Anthropologists have described reactions of Hopi Indians to death, mourning practices among the Cocopa Indians along the Mexican–American border, death and grief in Great Britain, the death culture of Mexican–Americans, relations between living Lugbara of East Africa and their ancestors and ghosts, and details of the death of a woman in a poverty-stricken Mexican family.[10-15] Other researchers have made cross-cultural comparisons of such phenomena as treatment of the aged and reactions to death, solutions to the problems of widowhood, funeral practices and burial rites.[16-19] Social scientists have written accounts of life in groups in which the elderly remain valued and active members, receive loving care when incapacitated and exhibit open acceptance of death.[20] These customs contrast with those becoming prevalent in Western society, in which old persons often live out their last years in a nursing home suffering both social stigma and social aversion.

PREPARATION FOR WORK WITH DYING PERSONS FROM DIFFERENT CULTURES

People are shaped by the cultural values of the ethnic, religious and social segment of the society in which they are reared. Persons who have grown to adulthood within "the context of a coherent culture" possess "an extraordinarily fine interlocking network of interpretations and conceptualizations" with which they encounter their "human and natural environment."[21] Thus attitudes toward death are not isolated phenomena but attributes closely linked to the whole complex of experience. For nurses, that experience has been further molded by their professional education.

Before they can become aware of and try to understand the ways in which members of other cultures view death and dying, nurses need to probe their own attitudes toward death and the basic assumptions that prevail in their local culture. When care givers closely examine some of the stressful events commonly associated with death and dying, they may find that many of these experiences are

As they explore their own feelings about death, nurses may become aware of personal beliefs and response patterns that are detrimental to themselves or to others.

laden with cultural expectations that can be reassessed, perhaps altered. As they explore their own feelings about death, nurses may become aware of personal beliefs and response patterns that are detrimental to themselves or to others.

Death in America

During the past 150 years, lower mortality rates and longer life expectancy have made death less visible, less meaningful and less controllable than it was in the past.[22] For many Americans, death has been "transposed, insulated, technologized, decontextualized."[23] As a youth-oriented society, Americans "transpose death from an immediate and perceptual menace to a distant remote prospect."[24] They insulate themselves from the death-dying sequence, turn their sick over to the hands of licensed experts and expect that

4

technology will be able to provide answers for all problems, including death.

Death has been lifted from its context in a reliable, tightly knit social fabric into the realm of personal decisions, which are frequently subject to decrees by experts and institutions. Nevertheless, some dying people and their families find ways to rebel against dying and grieving in what physicians, nurses and hospitals consider to be "the correct and most therapeutic style."[25]

Awareness of reactions to American mores

People from other cultures may be surprised or appalled by features of the American way of life. For example, the Bakongo of Zaïre want to return to their home village before they die. After death, the body is prepared for burial by close kin. These people would be horrified at the thought of dying miles from their natal village and leaving the preparation of the body in the hands of strangers as Americans do. Some deaths among the Bakongo might be termed homicides as there are frequent reports of sorcery and poisoning; however, suicide appears to be rare among these people. Consequently, the staff at a hospital in Zaïre were greatly shocked when an expatriate committed suicide there.[26]

Cross-cultural understanding is a two-way communication process that is often surprising and baffling to both sides. For example, beliefs about acceptable burial methods may differ radically from one culture to another. The Bakongo place the corpse in a rough, wooden coffin, bury it in the ground and may later erect a cement tombstone at the grave. The widow of an American who had been buried in Zaïre made arrangements that upon her death in the United States, her body would be cremated and the ashes deposited at her husband's grave. Since cremation is not practiced by the Bakongo, the arrival of a container of ashes and the accompanying instructions provoked considerable consternation.

Cultural sensitivity

Cultural sensitivity has several facets for nursing professionals:
- the feeling of respect for ethnic people of color as individuals and for their culture;
- the recognition that such people have cultural health beliefs and practices;
- the practice of modifying and improving nursing care to incorporate those beliefs and practices that are not life-threatening; and
- the ability to act on behalf of an ethnic client who is being denied safe and quality health care.[27]

Customs pertaining to language, food habits, religious practices, kinship structures, music and movement, manner of dress, standards for modesty, reactions to fear, responses to pain, and so forth, are learned, shared and transmitted from one generation to another. Experiences that run counter to accepted cultural norms may provoke feelings of distress that range from a vague sense of uneasiness or simple physical discomfort to rage, embarrassment or disgust.[28,29] Persons who resist medical or nursing regimens may be acting out of their cultural realities rather than from a tendency to be "difficult," "uncooperative" or "perverse."[30]

When caring for clients of different cultures than their own, nurses should be alert to the role of cultural conditioning in their own personal biases as well as in the response patterns of their clients. These biases are fostered through cultural stereotypes, that is, through reducing all people of a given culture to one mold and, thereby, disregarding the uniqueness and variability of individuals within that culture. In a candid but humorous account of his stay in a New York hospital, a Vietnamese professional man exposes this process as he recounts the derogatory labels, insensitive comments and inappropriate assessments made to and about him by the staff.[31]

In spite of the dangers of cultural stereotyping, medical workers can use careful generalizations when relating to clients. For example, each American Indian tribe has a unique language and different customs, but they share many core health beliefs.[32]

Factors relevant to terminal care of persons of different cultures

Communication

Communication, especially as expressed in language, is a major area of conflict and misunderstanding in any intercultural situation.[33,34] Persons who are ill may become depressed, distraught or terrified if they are unable to express their needs or understand instructions in the language used by care givers. Even if they have gained some facility in the language, they may be frustrated or embarrassed because of their accent or the unwillingness of others to try to understand them. Those who have learned other languages often lose a grasp of them and revert to their mother tongue during severe mental illness or as death approaches.[35,36]

Culture influences the forms of responses in conversation. For example, in the clinic situation, a Hispanic person may give a lengthy reply to a question, whereas an Asian client may simply answer yes or no. Both persons are following the norms of their culture: the former is careful to situate symptoms in the context of the environment; the latter refrains from divulging personal information to strangers.[37] To avoid giving a direct and painful no as a response to a request, a Filipino may use a hesitant yes or remain silent.[38]

Culture also affects the function of silence in conversation. "For a stranger entering an alien society, a knowledge of when *not* to speak may be as basic . . . as a knowledge of what to say."[39] For example, Western Apache Indians "give up on words" (keep silent) for varying intervals in situations in which relationships are ambiguous or unpredictable (e.g., when meeting strangers, in initial stages of courtship, in reunions with children who have been away at school, when "getting cussed out," when being with persons who are sad and when being with someone in a curing ceremonial.[40]

Affect and approach differ across cultures. For American Indians, calling attention to oneself is considered "showy" and inappropriate.[41] Samoan people consider themselves to be strong, able to take hardships without complaint and to bear up well under pain, calamities and death—in short, to be stoical.[42] A Filipino professional woman who has lived in the United States for several years shared the perceptions of her family and friends about

6

health care providers: Anglo nurses affect a cold, professional stance; Filipino nurses show warmth, display a personal and humane attitude and tend to humor and "tease" their patients to encourage compliance with treatment regimens.

Culture influences which topics are appropriate for conversation. American health care professionals are urged to engage in "more honest communication and sharing of information with dying patients" and are given instruction in doing so.[43,44] By contrast, the same Filipino woman mentioned above stated emphatically that in her culture the family and physician should reassure and "shelter" the patient from a bad prognosis. News of impending death would only add to the burden of the suffering one, so it is an act of mercy to spare the patient.

In the Arabic East, there is "substantial reluctance" on the part of physicians to share correct diagnoses with their patients.[45] In the Anglo culture, individuals tend to be euphemistic and circumspect when talking to a bereaved person about the loss of a loved one. Because they do not wish to provoke emotional outbursts, Americans treat grief "almost like an embarrassing disease."[46]

Within the Filipino culture, on the other hand, people often ask many specific factual questions of the bereaved and expect overt emotional responses to grief.

Because they do not wish to provoke emotional outbursts, Americans treat grief "almost like an embarrassing disease."

In the Jewish tradition, those who are making condolence visits are advised to enter the house and sit silently unless mourners show a desire to speak of their loss.[47] In some Native-American cultures, memory of the dead is suppressed, and people only speak of them with great reluctance.[48,49]

Values

All human groups face certain crucial issues: the character of innate human nature, the relation of the individual to nature and the supernatural, the relation of the person to other persons, and orientations toward time, activity and space. In facing these issues, people adopt distinctive value orientations that are in line with the basic tenets of their group.[50] Attitudes toward death and dying have been contrasted along these value orientations.[51]

Values may conflict sharply across cultural lines. For example, noninterference is a prime value of Native-Americans; intervention and coercion are fundamental elements of most Anglo groups.[52] Many other tribal and cultural values of American Indians are in direct contrast with those of the urban-industrial segment of society.[53]

Within the Filipino culture, great emphasis is placed on smooth interpersonal relationships, which are achieved through euphemisms, use of go-betweens and a "willingness to concede gracefully."[54] In the Mexican-American context, "respect" is a strong conservative force, especially when planning for a "proper" funeral. Family decisions are shaped by respect for elders, for tradition, for authority and for religion.[55] Within the Samoan community, reciprocity is a key value. During death or crisis, Samoans can count strongly on financial help, comfort and practical assistance from relatives, friends and even acquaintances who have moved away from the community. Those who receive help will in turn help others who are in distress.[56]

Orientation to time may be reflected in attitudes toward death and dying. In American culture, the future is cherished above the present or the past; time is viewed as finite, as a commodity to be redeemed lest it be irretrievably lost. From such a perspective, the elderly are often devalued as part of the past; the end of life is frequently feared as extermination that severs one from all that is meaningful.[57]

In contrast with Americans' view, Native-Americans see the universe as a harmonious whole in which human beings are part of the natural order and one with nature. Death is part of the normal pattern of life, an event to be accepted like the changing of the seasons.[58] Thus the American Indian prefers to take each day as it comes and live it to the fullest without fretting about the future or ruminating about death.[59] The Amish people also feel an affinity with nature and work with the seasons, not by the clock. For them, too, death is an expected part of life, an event to be faced with realism and equanimity.[60]

Concept of the family

The concept of "family" has different meanings across cultures. To Anglos, "family" usually refers to the nuclear family of mother, father and children. To Blacks and Hispanics, the term extends beyond parents and children to include grandparents, uncles, aunts, cousins, nieces, nephews and others. Spanish-speaking people may also refer to the children's godparents as part of the family.

Knowledge of cultural differences in kinship terms and in role expectations is important for care givers. For example, if they are not aware of these factors, non-Indian medical personnel may be puzzled by the arrival of several "mothers" at the bedside of a Native-American patient or by the presence of an Indian grandmother who takes primary responsibility for a child whose parents put in only occasional appearances at the hospital.[61]

Different cultural priorities may modify the degree to which families are involved in treatment regimens. Among Mexican-Americans, illness of a family member is a family affair.[62] Unlike a Western physician, who attends chiefly to the signs and symptoms of an individual, an Indian medicine man often treats the entire family along with the sick person.[63] Among Gypsies, the illness of one person may throw the whole family into a crisis; relatives accompany the sick one to the hospital and insist on remaining there regardless of regulations about visiting hours.[64]

Many terminally ill persons prefer to be at home to die in familiar surroundings under the care of their families. Mexican-Americans are often horrified at the common American practice of sending aged relatives to nursing homes when they become ill or senile.[65] To many people, hospitals and sanatoriums are fearful places.

Poor rural Blacks often look upon admission to a hospital as an indication of impending death.[66] Some older Blacks believe that "troublesome patients" in hospitals are poisoned and killed.[67] Chinese-Americans may fear that hospitals are not clean, that many people die there and that the spirits of these people get lost and are unable to find the way home.[68] Elderly Native-Americans may equate hospital admission with transfer to a funeral home. Beneath much of this apprehension is the fear of dying alone, of not having the solace of the family during the last hours.[69]

The desire to be with dying family members may be linked to religious beliefs. Many Native-Americans believe that the spirit of a dying person cannot leave the body until the family is there.[70] But gradually, even for American Indians, death is becoming impersonal as care is transferred from its familial context to the hospital and funeral home.[71] According to the customs of Orthodox Jews, relatives must remain with a dying family member so that the soul does not leave while the person is alone.[72] Jews do not leave a dead body unattended, as that would be a sign of disrespect.[73]

Cultural factors influence beliefs about communicating with children about death. In modern, mainstream America, children and young adults are usually shielded from contact with death. Today, many Americans reach the age of 35 before experiencing the death of close relatives or intimate friends. They are often without coping mechanisms that used to be acquired when people were cared for and died at home.

Among some segments of the American population, death is still highly visible and openly discussed. According to one study, death denial, avoidance and invisibility are not the norm in Kentucky; on the contrary, openness about death may be the dominant style there.[74] Furthermore, among such groups as Samoans, Amish, American Indians and Mexican-Americans, children help to care for dying relatives, attend funerals and take part in mourning practices.[75-78]

Religious beliefs

For many people, religious beliefs provide meaning for life and death. Suffering, illness and death are often conceived of as coming from God and requiring submission to His will.[79-81]

Many Spanish-speaking people view illness and pain as punishment from God for evil deeds or moral indiscretions. Feeling that they must accept suffering in order to atone for their sins, they may refuse pain relievers and nursing care and may engage in various types of penance.[82,83] Some of the practices of Mexican-Americans probably trace back to Mexican "home culture," with its elaborate concern with death and its traditional religious celebrations, such as the Days of the Dead.[84]

Many Blacks have a strong religious orientation that has helped them to survive against desperate odds. In the past, Black spirituals, poetry and literature were regarded as literal expressions of a longing to escape to the glorious freedom of the afterworld. Recently, it has been argued that traditional literature veiled a covert desire for freedom in this present world and communicated a secular view of death. In this perspective, practicality

Open discussion of death, care of dying family members at home and a high ceremonial emphasis on the death event help Amish people to cope with impending loss.

emerges as a prime value that assures a pragmatic distribution of scarce resources.[85,86] Furthermore, Black funerals, wakes and church social services provide psychosocial mechanisms that facilitate grief work.[87]

Deep religious faith and strong emotional ties contribute to a calm acceptance of death within the Amish community. Open discussion of death, care of dying family members at home and a high ceremonial emphasis on the death event help Amish people to cope with impending loss.[88]

Attitudes toward the body

Although pain is basically a physiological phenomenon, the meaning of pain and responses to it are subject to cultural prescription.[89] A study of hospital patients of Irish, Jewish, Italian and "Old American" origins revealed significant differences in attitudes and reactions toward pain. Similar responses appeared to mask underlying differences in attitudes toward pain and in the functions served by pain in various cultures.[90]

Concepts of modesty also vary from one culture to another. Among Hispanics, custom dictates that one must be modest when bathing, dressing, urinating and defecating, even when all others present are of the same sex.[91,92] Gypsies exhibit "great female genital modesty."[93] Muslims extend concern for modesty to care of the body after death. A male body is washed by male family members whenever possible; otherwise, the task may be done by the man's widow or by a woman who by Islamic tradition was ineligible to have married him. A female body is washed by female relatives or other women; the female body cannot be touched by any male, not even the dead woman's husband.[94]

Beliefs about the body influence attitudes toward such practices as transfusions, transplants and autopsies. In the Islamic view, a Muslim does not own his body; he holds it in a "sort of trust from God."[95] Consequently, a Muslim cannot donate or receive transplants of organs, and transfusions are only permissible if they are needed to save a person from death and if they are recommended by a physician who is a Muslim. The dead body must be buried intact; the autopsy rate is extremely low in Arab countries.[96] Physicians are not permitted to use cadavers for teaching or research purposes.[97]

Jews regard the body as a creation of God and the dwelling place of the soul; the body, whether living or dead, must be accorded great respect. Under Jewish law, many complex problems surround the question of organ transplants. Where live donors are involved (e.g., in kidney transplants), some rabbinic authorities rule that a transplant is permissible "if the probability of saving the recipient's life is substantially greater than the risk to the donor's life or health."[98] The major problem in heart transplants is the establishment of

10

the death of the donor.[99] Jewish law mandates abortion if the mother's life is at stake but prohibits it for any other reason.[100] Orthodox Jews regard autopsy as severe desecration of the body and forbid it unless suspicious circumstances surround the death or there is *immediate* possibility of saving another life. Liberal Jews do not object to autopsy; the decision is left to the family.[101]

Other religious and ethnic groups have varying attitudes toward amputations and autopsies. Hindus and Sikhs from India and Buddhists from India, Burma, Japan, Sri Lanka, Thailand, Vietnam and other Asian countries usually do not object to autopsies. Many Africans and West Indians are opposed to postmortem examinations.[102] Many American Indians view the dead body as a seed that is being placed in the ground. As a seed is planted whole, so the body should be buried intact; the idea of autopsy is repugnant.

If surgery must be performed, many Native-Indians want to reclaim the amputated limb or excised organ for proper burial at the time of removal or for storage in a freezer for burial with the body at the time of death. This precaution ensures that the individual is buried as a complete being and does not need to return after death.

Beliefs about the body also influence burial practices. Traditional Judaism is opposed to embalming and cremation; Jewish law requires burial of the body in the ground as soon as possible. Muslims wrap the body of the deceased in special pieces of cloth and bury it without a coffin in an earthen grave. According to Muslim law, a living person may not be put into fire even for punishment; so out of respect for the human being, a corpse may not be cremated.[103] The Roman Catholic Church traditionally prohibited cremation, but this ruling was recently revoked.[104] Attitudes toward disposition of the body varied among American Indians: Tlingit cremated their dead; Sioux exposed the body on funeral platforms; Pueblo buried their dead in the ground.[105] Quechan Indians still cremate their dead.[106]

Attitudes toward death

In some cultures, people believe that particular signs warn of approaching death. Many of these omens have to do with dreams or the appearance of an owl.[107-109] Death may also be attributed to breaking a taboo: an example of this was an incident in which nurses caring for an elderly American Indian patient removed her necklace and its attached curative objects and placed them with other personal items away from the bedside.[110]

Voodoo beliefs and practices still exist in the United States.[111] Incidents of sudden death following hexing or minor injuries have been attributed to various mechanisms: (1) the power of suggestion and total social isolation, which trigger fatal physiological responses,[112] (2) the giving-up–given-up complex[113] and (3) sensitization or tuning of the autonomic nervous system.[114]

Acceptance of sudden, violent death is problematic in most societies. Suicide is strictly forbidden under Islamic law. In the Filipino culture, suicide is shameful and brings disrepute on the whole family. Among Northern Cheyenne Indians, a "bad death" (usually as a result of a violent accident) disturbs the spiritual balance of the individual. This prevents sufficient reintegration to enable the self to find the way "over there," and condemns it to earthbound wanderings.[115]

For Blacks during the time of slavery or in present-day ghettos, death has often been sudden and harsh. Under these circumstances, violent death appears to create more open emotional outbursts and feelings of anger and rage than does natural or accidental death or suicide.[116]

Bereavement, grief and mourning practices

Bereavement is a sociological term indicative of the status and role of the survivor of a death. Differing family systems may ease or exacerbate the painful changes that bereaved persons experience. In the typical small nuclear family of Americans, in which the same few individuals fill most of the roles, death of one or more family members leaves a great void. By contrast, among Samoan immigrants to the United States, households often contain several generations. Within these extended families, the acute trauma of bereavement is muted by the fact that social roles of the deceased may be readily filled by other relatives. Furthermore, widowed persons usually remarry fairly soon, and new family ties are forged. Amish people also have multigenerational households and a high rate of remarriage after death of a spouse.

As an affective response to loss or death, the experience of grief is probably universal, but its expression is strongly influenced by cultural factors. When observing grief reactions in different family systems, a basic question needs to be asked: Who mourns for whom? Responses vary according to the lines of emotional attachment. For example, among the Ifaluk of Micronesia, a wife was not allowed or expected to grieve for her husband. Within that matrilineal society, a woman's emotional ties remained with male members of her maternal family; she was expected to grieve for her father, her brothers or her sons, but not for her spouse.[117]

Mourning is the culturally patterned behavioral response to a death.[118] Some

---

In the Jewish tradition, there are five successive stages of mourning; these stages extend over a year and include laws and practices that impinge on every aspect of life.

---

mourning rituals are highly structured and of long duration; others are fairly simple and relatively short. In the Jewish tradition, there are five successive stages of mourning; these stages extend over a year and include laws and practices that impinge on every aspect of life.[119]

For Northern Cheyennes, death of a relative or close friend brings deep and acute loneliness—the hardest experience that a human being has to bear. Grief is expected and tears are abundant, but weeping must cease in four days. Survivors must continue to live and find ways to cope with the exquisite pain of loneliness and isolation from the departed one.[120]

Among Quechan Indians, family and friends cry copiously during four days of

12

mourning. These tears are for the bereaved, not for the deceased; those who remain must somehow carry on, but the dead person is now happy because the pain and the struggle of this life have been left behind. After the cremation ceremony, the family return to their daily rounds and never speaks again of the deceased.[121]

Each culture has its own way of expressing grief. Some societies organize their recognition of bereavement around an effort to help the bereaved control themselves and forget; other societies direct their efforts toward helping survivors express and live out their grief.[122]

Funeral practices

Customs for disposal of the body after death vary widely. Muslims have specific rituals for washing, dressing and positioning the dead body.[123] Jews strongly discourage cosmetic restoration and viewing of the body or any attempt to hasten or retard decomposition by artificial means.[124] As part of their lifelong preparation for death, Amish women sew their own white burial garments as well as those of their family.[125]

Navajo fear to touch a body after death; they believe that the spirit or ghost of the dead person is contaminating. In preparation for burial, the body is dressed in fine apparel, adorned with expensive jewelry and money and wrapped in new blankets. After death, the Navajo must burn the structure in which the person died.[126] Among the Tlingit, family members exhibited a great unwillingness to touch the corpse. Often the dying person was dressed in funeral clothes several days before death occurred. By contrast, Siouan tribes showed no fear of the corpse; family members prepared the body for burial.[127]

Funeral arrangements vary from simple rituals to elaborate displays. Amish people rely upon family members, neighbors and friends for most of the support for their quiet ceremonies. Jewish families downplay materialistic concerns, use unadorned coffins and stress simplicity in burial services.[128] By contrast, there are reports that economically hard-pressed Navajo, Italian and Black families provide lavish and costly funerals.[129,130]

REFLECTIONS FOR NURSES

In both personal and professional life, nurses in the United States today frequently interact with people who subscribe to beliefs and practice lifeways that are very different from their own. To bridge this gap, health care professionals must become aware of and ready to identify and explore these differences. When in contact with persons of other cultures, nurses have an opportunity to turn every experience of difference and discomfort into a learning situation.[131]

Tools are available to enhance the learning possibilities in intercultural contacts. A few anthropologists have dared to recount their own successes and failures, their fortuitous advances and their maladroit overtures as they tried to gain entry into a new community and to understand a different culture.[132,133] A nurse-anthropologist has written of potential contributions of anthropology to nursing, particularly through the methodologies of participant-observation and ethnoscience.[134] In a guide for health care professionals who work with people of other cultures, a social scientist has formulated questions appropriate for every facet of medical care, including death and dying.[135] These queries are arranged under useful headings for the clinician: "What to find out," "Why it's important" and "How to do it."

But competent nursing care requires more than access to useful tools: it demands a commitment to helping clients and their families as they try to realize life and death experiences that are in accordance with their personal and cultural values. To function on this level, nurses must cultivate cultural sensitivity, that is, respect for individuals, recognition of their cultural health beliefs, incorporation of these practices insofar as possible into care plans and advocacy on behalf of ethnic clients.[136]

As they strive to provide appropriate care for persons who view life and death from different perspectives, health care professionals can counteract the seemingly relentless shift to depersonalization and dehumanization in our increasingly technologized society. In the process, nurses will find their own lives enriched and enhanced as understanding replaces fear and suspicion and strangers become friends.

REFERENCES

1. Murillo-Rohde, I. "Unique Needs of Ethnic Minority Clients in a Multiracial Society: A Socio-Cultural Perspective" in *Affirmative Action: Toward Quality Nursing Care for a Multiracial Society* ANA Pub. No. M-24 2500 (Kansas City: American Nurses' Association 1976) p. 26.

2. Myeroff, B. "Aging and the Aged in Other Cultures: An Anthropological Perspective" in Bauwens, E., ed. *The Anthropology of Health* (Saint Louis: C. V. Mosby 1978) p. 153.

3. Hiebert, P. *Cultural Anthropology* (Philadelphia: Lippincott 1976) p. 25.

4. Kalish, R., ed. *Death and Dying: Views from Many Cultures* (Farmingdale, N.Y.: Baywood—Perspectives on Death and Dying Series 1, 1980) p. 46.

5. Moore, J. "The Death Culture of Mexico and Mexican Americans" in Kalish, R., ed. *Death and Dying: Views from Many Cultures* (Farmingdale, N.Y.: Baywood—Perspectives on Death and Dying Series 1, 1980) p. 78.

6. Simmons, L. *The Role of the Aged in Primitive Society* (New Haven, Conn.: Yale University Press 1945) p. 244.

7. Racy, J. "Death in an Arab Culture." *Annals of the New York Academy of Sciences* 164:3 (1969) p. 871-880.

8. Tichauer, R. "Attitudes Toward Death and Dying Among the Aymara Indians of Bolivia." *Journal of the American Medical Women's Association* 19:6 (1964) p. 463-466.

9. Daynes, G. "Intercultural Problems in the Care of the Dying Patient." *South African Medical Journal* 48:4 (1974) p. 140.

10 Kennard, E. "Hopi Reactions to Death." *American Anthropologist* 39:3 (1937) p. 491-496.

11. Kelly, W. "Cocopa Attitudes and Practices with Respect to Death and Mourning." *Southwestern Journal of Anthropology* 5:2 (1949) p. 151-164.

12. Gorer, G. *Death, Grief, and Mourning* (New York: Doubleday 1965).

13. Moore. "The Death Culture of Mexico and Mexican Americans." p. 72-91.

14. Middleton, J. "The Cult of the Dead: Ancestors and Ghosts" in Lessa, W. and Vogt, E., eds. *Reader in Comparative Religion* 3rd ed. (New York: Harper & Row 1972) p. 487-492.

15. Lewis, O. *A Death in the Sanchez Family* (New York: Random House 1969).

16. Simmons. *The Role of the Aged in Primitive Society.*

17. Mathison, J. "A Cross-Cultural View of Widowhood." *Omega* 1:3 (1970) p. 201-218.

18. Pine, V. "Comparative Funeral Practices." *Practical Anthropology* 16:2 (1969) p. 49-62.

19. Bendann, E. *Death Customs: An Analytical Study of Burial Rites* (New York: Knopf 1966).

20. Reid, J., Yunupingu, L. and Yunupingu, D. "Caring for the Aged and Dying in an Australian Aboriginal

14

Community." *Australasian Nurses Journal* 7:2 (1978) p. 26.

21. Bateson, M. "Insight in a Bicultural Context." *Philippines Studies* 16:4 (1968) p. 606.

22. Krant, M. *Dying and Dignity: The Meaning and Control of a Personal Death* (Springfield, Ill.: Charles C. Thomas 1974) p. 6.

23. Kastenbaum, R. and Aisenberg, R. *The Psychology of Death* (New York: Springer 1972) p. 205.

24. Ibid. p. 206.

25. Taylor, C. "Death, American Style." *Death Education* 1:2 (1977) p. 177.

26. Ross, M. Personal experience in the Republic of Zaïre 1961-1974.

27. Bello, T. "The Third Dimension: Cultural Sensitivity in Nursing Practice." *Imprint* 23:1 (1976) p. 36.

28. Hall, E. *The Silent Language* (Greenwich, Conn.: Fawcett 1959).

29. Hall, E. *The Hidden Dimension* (Garden City, N.Y.: Anchor 1966).

30. MacGregor, F. "Uncooperative Patients: Some Cultural Interpretations" in Brink, P., ed. *Transcultural Nursing: A Book of Readings* (Englewood Cliffs, N.J.: Prentice-Hall 1976) p. 37.

31. Tao-Kim-Hai, A. "Orientals Are Stoic" in MacGregor, F. *Social Science in Nursing: Applications for the Improvement of Patient Care* (New York: Russell Sage Foundation 1960) p. 313-326.

32. Primeaux, M. "American Indian Health Care Practices: A Cross-Cultural Perspective." *Nursing Clinics of North America* 12:1 (1977) p. 64.

33. Hall, E. and Whyte, W. "Intercultural Communication: A Guide to Men of Action." *Human Organization* 19:1 (1960) p. 5-12.

34. Riffenburgh, R. "Communication in Cross-Cultural Medical Practice." *Western Medicine* 7:11 (1966) p. 320-322.

35. Leininger, M. *Nursing and Anthropology: Two Worlds to Blend* (New York: John Wiley & Sons 1970) p. 86-94.

36. Daynes. "Intercultural Problems in the Care of the Dying Patient." p. 139.

37. Bello. "The Third Dimension: Cultural Sensitivity in Nursing Practice." p. 38.

38. Parreno, H. "How Pilipinos Deal with Stress." *Washington State Journal of Nursing* 49:1 (1977) p. 5.

39. Basso, K. " 'To Give Up on Words': Silence in Western Apache Culture." *Southwestern Journal of Anthropology* 26:3 (1970) p. 215.

40. Ibid. p. 216-225.

41. Primeaux. "American Indian Health Care Practices: A Cross-Cultural Perspective." p. 93.

42. Ablon, J. "Bereavement in a Samoan Community."

British Journal of Medical Psychology 44:4 (1971) p. 382.

43. Feifel, H. "Death and Dying in Modern America." *Death Education* 1:1 (1977) p. 14.

44. Benoliel, J. "Talking to Patients About Death." *Nursing Forum* 9:3 (1970) p. 254-268.

45. Racy. "Death in an Arab Culture." p. 874.

46. Bateson. "Insight in a Bicultural Context." p. 612.

47. Chafetz, P. "Jewish Practices in Death and Mourning." *Death Education* 3:4 (1980) p. 367.

48. Kelly. "Cocopa Attitudes and Practices with Respect to Death and Mourning." p. 153.

49. Kennard. "Hopi Reactions to Death." p. 492.

50. Kluckhohn, F. and Strodtbeck, F. *Variations in Value Orientations* (Evanston, Ill.: Row, Peterson 1961) p. 11.

51. Spiegel, J. "Cultural Variations in Attitudes toward Death and Disease" in Grosser, G., Wechsler, H. and Greenblatt, M., eds. *The Threat of Impending Disaster* (Cambridge, Mass.: MIT Press 1964) p. 284-299.

52. Good Tracks, J. "Native American Non-interference." *Social Work* 18:6 (1973) p. 30-34.

53. Proctor, N. "Providing Services to American Indians: Interaction or Interference?" Mimeographed (Paper presented at the annual meeting of the American Psychological Association, New York City, 1979).

54. Parreno. "How Pilipinos Deal with Stress." p. 5.

55. Moore. "The Death Culture of Mexico and Mexican Americans." p. 80-90.

56. Ablon. "Bereavement in a Samoan Community." p. 329-338.

57. Myeroff. "Aging and the Aged in Other Cultures: An Anthropological Perspective." p. 158.

58. Dial, A. "Death in the Life of Native Americans." *Indian Historian* 11:3 (1978) p. 33.

59. Primeaux, M. "Caring for the American Indian Patient." *American Journal of Nursing* 77:1 (1977) p. 94.

60. Bryer, K. "The Amish Way of Death: A Study of Family Support Systems." *American Psychologist* 34:3 (1979) p. 255-261.

61. Primeaux. "American Indian Health Care Practices: A Cross-Cultural Perspective." p. 61.

62. Gonzales, H. "Health Care Needs of the Mexican-American" in *Ethnicity and Health Care* NLN Pub. No. 14-1625 (New York: National League for Nursing 1975) p. 24.

63. Primeaux. "American Indian Health Care Practices: A Cross-Cultural Perspective." p. 61.

64. Anderson, G. and Tighe, B. "Gypsy Culture and

Health Care." *American Journal of Nursing* 73:2 (1973) p. 284.

65. Clark, M. *Health and the Mexican-American Culture* 2nd ed. (Berkeley: University of California Press 1970) p. 145.

66. McCabe, G. "The Cultural Influences on Patient Care." *American Journal of Nursing* 60:8 (1960) p. 1103.

67. Martin, B. "Ethnicity and Health Care: Afro-Americans" in *Ethnicity and Health Care* NLN Pub. No. 14-1625 (New York: National League for Nursing 1975) p. 54.

68. Campbell, T. and Chang, B. "Health Care of the Chinese in America." *Nursing Outlook* 21:4 (1973) p. 249.

69. McCabe. "The Cultural Influences on Patient Care." p. 1103.

70. White, E. "Giving Health Care to Minority Patients." *Nursing Clinics of North America* 12:1 (1977) p. 32.

71. Dial. "Death in the Life of Native Americans." p. 36.

72. Berkowitz, P. and Berkowitz, N. "The Jewish Patient in the Hospital." *American Journal of Nursing* 67:11 (1967) p. 2337.

73. Rabinowicz, H. "The Jewish View of Death." *Nursing Times* 75:18 (1979) p. 757.

74. Garrity and Wyss. "Death, Funeral and Bereavement Practices in Appalachian and Non-Appalachian Kentucky." *Omega* 7:3 (1976) p. 226.

75. Ablon. "Bereavement in a Samoan Community." p. 226.

76. Bryer. "The Amish Way of Death: A Study of Family Support Systems." p. 259.

77. Dial. "Death in the Life of Native Americans." p. 36.

78. Moore. "The Death Culture of Mexico and Mexican Americans." p. 80.

79. Snow, L. "The Religious Component in Southern Folk Medicine." *The Conch* 8:1,2 (1976) p. 26-51.

80. Ablon. "Bereavement in a Samoan Community." p. 332.

81. Chafetz. "Jewish Practices in Death and Mourning." p. 365.

82. Murillo-Rohde. "Unique Needs of Ethnic Minority Clients in a Multiracial Society: A Sociocultural Perspective." p. 29.

83. Gonzales. "Health Care Needs of the Mexican-American." p. 23.

84. Green, J. "The Days of the Dead in Oaxaxa, Mexico: An Historical Inquiry" in Kalish, R., ed. *Death and Dying: Views from Many Cultures.* p. 56-71.

85. Jackson, M. "The Black Experience of Death" in Kalish, R., ed. *Death and Dying: Views from Many Cultures.* p. 97.

86. Kalish, R. and Reynolds, D. *Death and Ethnicity: A Psychocultural Study* (Los Angeles: University of Southern California Press 1976) p. 109.

87. Masamba, J. and Kalish, R. "Death and Bereavement: The Role of the Black Church." *Omega* 7:1 (1976) p. 30.

88. Bryer. " The Amish Way of Death: A Study of Family Support Systems." p. 255-261.

89. Saunders, L. "Culture and Nursing Care" in Jaco, E., ed. *Patients, Physicians and Illness* (Glencoe, Ill.: The Free Press 1958) p. 538.

90. Zborowski. "Cultural Components in Responses to Pain." *Journal of Social Issues* 8:4 (1952) p. 21-25.

91. Murillo-Rohde. "Unique Needs of Ethnic Minority Clients in a Multiracial Society: A Sociocultural Perspective." p. 32.

92. Gonzales. "Health Care Needs of the Mexican-American." p. 23.

93. Anderson and Tighe. "Gypsy Culture and Health Care." p. 261.

94. Baqui, A. "Muslim Teaching Concerning Death." *Nursing Times* 75:14 (April 5, 1979 Occasional Papers) p. 44.

95. Ibid.

96. Racy. "Death in an Arab Culture." p. 875.

97. Baqui. "Muslim Teaching Concerning Death." p. 44.

98. Rosner, F. "Organ Transplants: The Jewish Viewpoint." *Journal of Thanatology* 3:3/4 (1975) p. 238.

99. Ibid. p. 240.

100. Rotkovitch. "Ethnicity and Health Care—The Jewish Heritage." p. 42.

101. Berkowitz and Berkowitz. "The Jewish Patient in the Hospital." p. 2337.

102. Lally, M. "Last Rites and Funeral Customs of Minority Groups." *Midwife, Health Visitor, and Community Nurse* 14:7 (1978) p. 224-225.

103. Baqui. "Muslim Teaching Concerning Death." p. 44.

104. Formby, J. "Christian Teaching Concerning Death: A Roman Catholic Approach." *Nursing Times* 74:15 (1978 Occasional Papers) p. 59.

105. Dial. "Death in the Life of Native Americans." p. 35.

106. Swift Arrow, B. "Funeral Rites of the Quechan Tribe." *Indian Historian* 7:2 (1974) p. 24.

107. Craven, M. *I Heard the Owl Call My Name* (New York: Dell Publishing 1973).

108. Straus, A. "The Meaning of Death in Northern

16

Cheyenne Culture." *Plains Anthropologist: Journal of the Plains Conference* 23:79 (1978) p. 2.

109. Clark. *Health and the Mexican-American Culture.* p. 146.

110. Primeaux. "Caring for the American Indian Patient." p. 92.

111. Martin. "Ethnicity and Health Care: Afro-Americans." p. 53.

112. Cannon, W. " 'Voodoo' Death." *American Anthropologist* 44:2 (1942) p. 169-181.

113. Lester, D. "Voodoo Death: Some New Thoughts on an Old Phenomenon." *American Anthropologist* 74:3 (1972) p. 386-390.

114. Lex, B. "Voodoo Death: New Thoughts on an Old Explanation." *American Anthropologist* 76:4 (1974) p. 818-823.

115. Straus. "The Meaning of Death in Northern Cheyenne Culture." p. 3.

116. Masamba and Kalish. "Death and Bereavement: The Role of the Black Church." p. 33.

117. Fulton, R. "The Sociology of Death." *Death Education* 1:1 (1977) p. 16.

118. Reid, J. "A Time to Live; A Time to Grieve: Patterns and Processes of Mourning Among the Yolngu of Australia." *Culture, Medicine and Psychiatry* 3:4 (1979) p. 321.

119. Chafetz. "Jewish Practices in Death and Mourning." p. 366-369.

120. Straus. "The Meaning of Death in Northern Cheyenne Culture." p. 3-6.

121. Swift Arrow, B. "Funeral Rites of the Quechan Tribe." p. 22-24.

122. Bateson. "Insight in a Bicultural Context." p. 612.

123. Baqui. "Muslim Teaching Concerning Death." p. 43-44.

124. Chafetz. "Jewish Practices in Death and Mourning." p. 364-365.

125. Bryer. "The Amish Way of Death: A Study of Family Support Systems." p. 257.

126. French, J. and Schwartz, D. "Terminal Care at Home in Two Cultures." *American Journal of Nursing* 73:3 (1973) p. 503.

127. Dial. "Death in the Life of Native Americans." p. 35.

128. Gordon, A. "The Jewish View of Death: Guidelines for Mourning" in Kubler-Ross, E., ed. *Death: The Final Stage of Growth* (Englewood Cliffs, N.J.: Prentice-Hall 1975) p. 47.

129. French and Schwartz. "Terminal Care at Home in Two Cultures." p. 505.

130. McDonald, M. "The Management of Grief: A Study of Black Funeral Practices." *Omega* 4:2 (1973) p. 139-148.

131. Bateson. "Insight in a Bicultural Context." p. 607.

132. Powdermaker, H. *Stranger and Friend: The Way of an Anthropologist* (New York: Norton 1966).

133. Wax, R. *Doing Fieldwork: Warnings and Advice* (Chicago: University of Chicago Press 1971).

134. Leininger. *Nursing and Anthropology: Two Worlds to Blend.* p. 24-25; 167-178.

135. Brownlee, A. *Community, Culture, and Care: A Cross-cultural Guide for Health Workers* (Saint Louis: C. V. Mosby 1978).

136. Bello. "The Third Dimension: Cultural Sensitivity in Nursing Practice." p. 36.

Care of a hospitalized dying patient

Maureen Niland, RN, MS
Instructor, Nursing Education
Seattle Veterans Administration Medical
* Center*
Doctoral Student
University of Washington
Seattle, Washington

Judith Atwood, RN, MN
Clinical Supervisor/Specialist
Harbor View Medical Center

Clinical Assistant Professor
University of Washington
Seattle, Washington

KAREN, her husband and her six-month-old son arrived from out of town on a bright, sunny April day. They came to a recognized specialty medical center to cure Karen of moderately advanced choriocarcinoma, a rapidly progressive and potentially lethal type of cancer. During Karen's three-month hospitalization, the staff and Karen focused on the goal of cure, until less than 24 hours before her death.

For those providing her care, Karen was a remarkable young woman who motivated staff to use some nursing care concepts and approaches they had previously only read about in the professional literature. The approaches used included a primary nursing's examination of the differences between the principles and approaches of the care model and the

This article is adapted from Niland, M. and Atwood, J. "Contracting with Karen: A Patient with Trophoblastic Disease" in Peterson, B. H. and Kellogg, C. J., eds., Current Practice in Oncologic Nursing *(St. Louis: C.V. Mosby Co. 1976).*

0164-0534/81/0033-0017$2.00
© 1981 Aspen Systems Corporation

cure model as applied in Karen's situation, preservation of the patient's control over her life and contracting as a method of ensuring that essential care was given while Karen's dignity and life style were preserved.

Karen's goal of cure was congruent with that of the total staff and easily served as the overall framework for working with her until very late in her stay at the medical center. The ability of the patient, his or her family and the care givers to share a common frame of reference in the planning and implementation of care is central to the process of providing quality care. All concerned in this situation endured hard work, pain and the unpleasantness associated with the treatment of the cancer. But in the unified team, each member served to support the others' goal of cure. In retrospect, these experiences proved to be meaningful personally and professionally.

THE CURE MODEL VERSUS THE MAINTENANCE CARE MODEL

As part of the unified plan, the staff became particularly concerned about Karen's having control over and understanding the plan of care. For Karen to be committed to enduring the unpleasant aspects of obtaining a cure (essentially the side effects of treatment added to the toll taken by the disease), it became obvious that she needed to retain control over her daily activities. She also needed to understand enough of what was going on to turn the unknown into the known. The care givers, while operating in a cure model, had to recognize that the time could come when curing Karen would not be realistic. Therefore, the staff needed to be ready to switch with Karen to a maintenance care model.

In the maintenance care model, the patient usually cannot be cured by any modality currently known. It therefore becomes necessary to accept what is often perceived as second best: to help the patient die comfortably or live with a significant disability. The cure model is prevalent in the health care delivery system today despite recognition of the problems this approach can create for patients, families and staff.

Changing from a cure model to a care model, when appropriate, is still too rarely done. Many patients are afraid of being rejected if they do not adhere to health care professionals' need to cure. Some nurses and other professionals have difficulty providing for the care needs of a patient who is dying and direct their energies toward patients for whom the outcome is cure.

On the other hand, when the patient is oriented toward cure and the staff goal is not congruent, staff find themselves in a difficult situation. When this occurs, staff may encourage less patient adherence to the treatment regimen. If the patient, his or her family or the staff function exclusively

---

Although not the sole requirement for effective care, contracts with the health care staff helped Karen retain control, self-care and life-style activities until just prior to her death.

---

within one model—cure or maintenance care—the patient is afforded less control and self-direction. In Karen's situation, contracts were established with primary care givers. Although not the sole requirement for effective care, these contracts with the health care staff helped Karen retain control, self-care and life-style activities until just prior to her death.

KAREN

Karen was 23, pale, frightened and withdrawn when arriving at the medical center. She tired easily and at times was short of breath. Karen and her husband had been married for five years and seemed to have a close relationship. Both gave the impression of being private people. They had married after graduating from high school and continued to live in a small town. The trip to the medical center was the first major trip either had taken. Their income from Karen's husband's blue-collar job had been adequate, but he had to quit his job when they left their small town.

The previous September they had their first child. Two years previously, Karen had been pregnant for the first time and had passed a hydatidiform mole. Subsequently, she had no further signs of trophoblastic disease. Karen again became pregnant after waiting the required year. The pregnancy appeared normal, as was the delivery.

Five months later, Karen entered a local hospital, complaining of shortness of breath and shoulder and chest pain. She was diagnosed as having pneumonia, but she did not respond to therapy. She developed a pleural effusion, which when tapped, was negative for trophoblastic cells. Serum and urine human chorionic gonadotropin tests (HCGs) were then done. These tests were found positive, and Karen was diagnosed as having trophoblastic disease.

TROPHOBLASTIC DISEASE

Trophoblastic diseases have been classified in several ways. They are divided into those that are gestational neoplasms and arise from placental tissues and those that are nongestational neoplasms. Gestational trophoblastic disease includes hydatidiform mole and choriocarcinoma. Trophoblastic disease is considered metastatic if evidence of extrauterine growth can be found either in the pelvic cavity or elsewhere.

All trophoblastic diseases are uncommon. The hydatidiform mole is the most frequent and occurs in about 1 of every 1,500 to 2,500 pregnancies in the United States. About 5 percent of molar pregnancies progress to more advanced forms of the illness, and not all advanced forms of the illness come from a molar pregnancy.

Hydatidiform mole is a benign neoplasm confined to the uterus. Choriocarcinoma is usually characterized by a rapid proliferation of cells and early distant metastatic invasion. Early metastasis most commonly involves the lungs. Other target organs are the liver, brain, heart and kidneys. If untreated, metastatic trophoblastic disease (such as choriocarcinoma) is rapidly progressive and often fatal within a year. However, patients who begin chemotherapy less than four months after onset of the disease and patients with a urinary

20

HCG titer less than 10,000 I.U. have an excellent prognosis. Up to 98 percent of these patients are cured of the disease.[1]

The diagnosis of all forms of trophoblastic disease is established by finding characteristic elevations of the HCG titers in urine or plasma. Malignant trophoblastic disease is frequently diagnosed because of signs and symptoms of metastasis and a high degree of suspicion as to their origin. In Karen's situation, the above described "pneumonia" that did not respond to therapy was the first clue. In the face of Karen's history of a molar pregnancy, HCG levels were tested and found elevated, thus confirming the diagnosis.

At the time of her admission, Karen's condition did not fit into any of the following categories: (1) less than four months since onset of disease, (2) low HCG levels or (3) advanced disease. This was due to her prior chemotherapy and the difficulty in being sure that presumed side effects from this treatment were not signs of progressive disease. It was within this context that the decision to focus on curing Karen was established as a framework for her care. The lack of clear-cut prognostic expectations was, however, explicitly discussed. Once the cure decision was established, the tone for the care planning process was set.

PLANNING OF CARE

Karen's overall problem was limited physical energy, which resulted from the physiological problems of choriocarcinoma and its treatment. From Karen's point of view, it was important to be well groomed and vibrant when seeing her husband and child, to get well and to go home. Because of her limited energy, Karen's goals were at times difficult for her to achieve. Even though she got along well with the staff, her lack of energy made her resistive to care. Planning of care focused on curative therapy and ways of helping Karen conserve energy for maintenance of her physical functions and personal appearance.

Curative therapy

Chemotherapy, with a variety of drugs was the treatment used in an attempt to cure Karen. She received 5 days of treatment followed by a 14-day rest period, during which she recovered from some of the toxic effects of the drugs. This regimen was followed throughout her stay, with some variations in the time required for the rest periods.

Karen was carefully monitored through a variety of tests, including white blood cell counts, differential counts, platelet counts and liver and renal studies. The progress of the disease was monitored through weekly chest X-rays, selective brain studies and careful observation of her general condition.

Karen developed most of the signs of drug toxicity—particularly uncomfortable stomatitis and rashes. Her respiratory metastasis continued to develop, and other areas of metastasis began to appear. Nevertheless, she remained able to recover sufficiently from each new development of the disease to go on overnight passes and other family outings throughout her stay. Moreover, at the time of her death, she was far better able to walk, eat, groom herself to look attractive and participate in family life than the vast majority of people with her degree of illness.

Contracting

One of the major strategies used to maintain Karen's energy and ability for self-care was contracting. A contract is defined as "an agreement between two or more parties."[2] A contract may be formal or informal, written or verbal. Expectations and goals are made explicit for all persons involved in the contract. As a common frame of reference, a contract can draw together all health team members, including patient and family, for sharing in care and accomplishing goals of therapy.

Although some of the elements of contracting are found in other approaches, such as behavior modification, contracting differs from other approaches in that the patient's desires are included in the agreement. In contracting, the nurse and patient have "different but equal responsibilities toward common goals."[3]

The first step in drawing up a contract is to reach an agreement between significant members of the team (including the patient) who are the most directly involved in the care planning process. All involved in the care must be apprised of the agreements. In Karen's situation, four people were primarily responsible for establishing the contract. One nurse was designed as the primary nurse. This nurse worked with the physician specialist and resident, who were responsible for medical care.

Together, the primary nurse, the two primary physicians and Karen established the contractual agreements. Karen's husband was less involved because he chose to have limited direct involvement in her care. His energies were devoted to a local job, the care of their son and visits with Karen each evening. Karen assumed responsibility for integrating her husband into the plans.

Ideally, all of the persons involved in a contract should agree with its specifications; realistically, this is rarely the case. Therefore, disagreements must be successfully mediated. Primary health team members must find compromises, settle disputes and with the patient, alter the contract as needed. The patient should not be put in the negotiator position for team disputes. This activity needlessly consumes the patient's already limited energy.

A realistic appraisal of the situation may mean the patient will need to know when major differences in opinion occur and to understand the basis for the differences. Most patients find that such an honest approach decreases frustration and assists them in coping with minor contractual variations. Karen was able to effectively deal with variations in the contract. When conflicts arose or staff did not follow through on contractual agreements, the primary nurse usually assumed the negotiator role.

The major job of the patient in a contract is adherence to agreed-upon activities; for Karen, these activities varied

---

The major job of the patient in a contract is adherence to agreed-upon activities; for Karen, these activities varied with the phase of disease and treatment.

---

with the phase of disease and treatment. Steckel points out that reinforcers for adherence to a plan of care are quite individualistic.[4] For Karen, reinforcement for participation in daily activities centered around her appearance, particularly when she was with her husband, and going home on pass. When Karen managed her care well, she had a maximum level of energy for grooming, communicating with her husband during visits and being away from the hospital on pass.

KAREN'S PROBLEMS

During most of the three months that Karen was under care, her problems remained constant. Problem severity varied with the phase of the disease process and the treatment regimen. Although Karen's active involvement in care was altered according to the severity of her problems, she remained in control of her care.

Six problems emerged, all of which influenced Karen's energy level:

1. progress of the disease process and toxic responses to treatment;
2. pain and discomfort;
3. nutritional wasting;
4. immobility;
5. prevention of infection, especially respiratory; and
6. fear of dying.

Progress of the disease process and toxic responses to treatment

The combination of the disease, the toxic effects of chemotherapy and a concomitant decrease in Karen's overall energy level made it a real challenge to maintain her activity level and energy on a day-to-day basis. Maintaining her energy was particularly important to her, as one of her major goals was to be able to spend as much time as possible out of the hospital with her son and husband.

The greatest energy drains Karen experienced were caused by the truly unpleasant toxic side effects of the chemotherapy. Principal among these were pain, malaise and advanced stomatitis. The combination of these toxic effects made it difficult to impossible for her to retain enough motivation to engage in her normal self-care and grooming activities. The stomatitis and pain made it impossible for her to tolerate food and, at times, liquids; hence, it affected her nutritional state and further impaired her energy.

After the first two of her many courses of chemotherapy, it became evident that there was a pattern relating to how she felt and the chemotherapy/rest cycle of her treatment. Using this information, the nurses were able to negotiate a contract using a variable care plan based on the phase of her treatment. The essentials of the variable care plan appear in the boxed insert.

It was much easier for Karen to do well with activities of daily living (ADL) and usually with nutrition. However, she disliked the respiratory therapy and oral care and would bargain persistently for changes in these areas. Other areas of the contract were more difficult for Karen, especially those relating to discomfort and pain. The staff were able to come to satisfactory agreements with Karen.

Pain and discomfort

Through the use of contracting, Karen was afforded more control over her prob-

Karen's Variable Care Plan

Therapy and rest cycle	Toxic symptoms energy level	Contractual activity level
Therapy—5 days	Minimal symptoms, slightly lethargic	Self-care for all agreed-on activities
Rest period		
Day 1—after therapy	General malaise, discomfort, decreased energy	Activities of daily living, general hygiene, self-care
Day 2—after therapy	Specific symptoms appeared, very low energy	Minimum ADL and respiratory therapy; assisted care
Days 3 and 4—after therapy	All symptoms present, very uncomfortable, needed sedation/sleep	Light sedation, mouth care, IV, ADL (at least turn, cough, deep breath) Nurses gave care
Days 5-14—after therapy	Gradual return to minimal symptoms	All agreed-on activities
	Gradual return to normal energy	Self-care

lem with pain than most patients usually are given in a similar situation. The agreements made were the following: (1) Karen would gradually increase her self-management of medications for pain in the hospital; and (2) she could go home on pass if she successfully managed herself on oral pain medications when she had reached an established state of recovery from her treatment.

The primary nurse shared information with Karen regarding the effects of the pain medications and how these drugs could affect activities of daily living. She was told the drugs she could use and given information about the consequences of heavy sedation. After it was determined that Karen understood the effects of the drugs, she started selecting drugs according to the quality and quantity of her pain. As Karen increased her ability to manage her pain, she increased her control over the selection of the medications.

The medication objectives for Karen were for her to be comfortable and to maintain maximum functional ability. Inappropriate management, so that she received either too little medication for comfort or too heavy sedation, impaired her physical functioning ability, her personal appearance and her ability to participate fully in her relationship with her husband.

Karen was well motivated for good management of her medications. If she managed poorly, she had less control and more difficulty achieving her goals. At no time did Karen abuse the use of drugs. In fact, when she had primary responsibility for managing her pain, she used less of the potent medications than were given to her when she was managed by staff.

Some difficulties did arise in contracting with Karen in the management of her pain. Although Karen followed through on prior agreements, some staff members were philosophically unable to accept allowing a patient to have control over pain management. It was important for the staff and Karen to resolve this breach in contract and not perceive it as a reflection of good versus poor care. When incidents arose, the primary nurse discussed them with Karen and then with the staff. The focus was on how well Karen had done in attempting to manage her pain, not on the responses of staff members.

Nutritional wasting

Another problem that affected Karen's physical energy level and personal appearance was her nutritional status. This occurred because of the wasting process associated with choriocarcinoma as well as the side effects of drug therapy, especially stomatitis. Karen realized that sustaining her nutritional intake was important for helping to prevent wasting, and she was well motivated to maintain her weight because of her concern for her personal appearance. However, her discomfort from nausea and vomiting, and from gingivitis and stomatitis during and immediately after treatment, made this task difficult.

The nutritional goal for Karen was minimum weight loss through a plan that was acceptable to her. She lost a total of 12 pounds during her entire hospitalization. Some difficulty was encountered because Karen never fully agreed with all the care that staff members believed was necessary. This difficulty was resolved by settling on a minimum acceptable level of nutrition rather than the ideal. Three levels of nutritional intake were expected of Karen, depending on how she felt. While the lowest level did not meet her nutritional

needs, she made up for this, in large part, during her best phases.

Oral care for stomatitis required the greatest compromise. When the stomatitis was at its worst, Karen usually resisted oral care. Her mouth was so sore that her own secretions caused her discomfort, and water was intolerable. Local anesthetics did not provide relief; the discomfort from application of the local anesthetic greatly outweighed any relief achieved.

Various types of oral care were tried, but Karen's response to them was poor. The staff accepted the fact that Karen would do no oral care during her worst periods. This situation was less than desirable, but after bargaining, this limited care was accepted as the maximum Karen would allow. Karen did manage well in other areas of care during her worst periods. She bargained for oral care to be one area in which she would receive what staff believed was minimum care.

Immobility

Immobility was a problem that lent itself with great ease to contracting. The goal was maximum physical functioning considering all previously stated problems. Thus how well other problems were managed directly influenced mobility. After receiving instructions, Karen was able to choose the activities she would perform in relation to the severity of her toxicity pattern. Although she needed encouragement, she was able to follow through on the agreements.

On her best days, Karen took complete care of herself. On her bad days (except a few when she was severely toxic), activities were adjusted accordingly, but she still carried out essential activities of daily living. This plan was successful from both Karen's and the staff's point of view.

Prevention of infection, especially respiratory

Negotiating care to prevent infection was difficult. One reason may have been that prevention was a staff goal, and Karen never really internalized it as a problem. Furthermore, some of the measures to prevent infection caused her discomfort. In addition to prevention of infection associated with her stomatitis, prevention of respiratory infection was essential.

A respiratory therapy program was developed using rebreathers and a positive pressure ventilator to encourage adequate chest expansion. The use of the equipment and taking deep breaths were uncomfortable for Karen during her worst days, and compromises in her schedule were worked out. As Karen improved, she was supposed to assume responsibility for her own respiratory care. She was given cards for the times of respiratory therapy. This approach was helpful, but she still required much reminding to follow through.

It is interesting to note that Karen never forgot to take her birth control pills, but she usually forgot to do the respiratory therapy. Fortunately, Karen never developed any significant infections, at least none requiring antibiotic therapy. As it turned out, both the staff and Karen had to compromise in the area of respiratory care, and the staff compromised on care for stomatitis.

Fear of dying

During the majority of Karen's stay, the fear of dying was an underlying problem, infrequently dealt with primarily because of the focus on cure. Twenty-four hours before Karen died, dying suddenly emerged as the dominant problem.

KAREN'S DEATH

The onset of the terminal phase of Karen's illness was insidious. During the last month of her life, she gradually began to show increasing signs that the disease was progressing. HCG levels became resistant, signs indicating increasing respiratory disability became more obvious and she bounced back very slowly from the side effects of the chemotherapy. The energy Karen previously devoted to maintaining her appearance declined. She showed subtle signs of a slipping commitment to the cure goal. For example, previously, both Karen and her primary nurse established concrete and specific criteria for her activities of daily living, but during the last month, both began to "go through the motions," and the criteria became more general.

No one talked about how Karen was doing. Anxiety began to be manifested in short tempers and other such behaviors. This climate had just begun to settle in when Karen had a grand mal seizure. Anxiety among the staff became overt, and they began to make such statements as "the game is being lost" or even "unless a miracle happens, Karen might die." Karen asked for confirmation of what she knew intuitively: the seizure was a strong indication that the cancer had metastasized to the brain. Karen and the rest of the team began the process of switching from a cure model to a maintenance care model.

26

Immediately after the seizure, the shift from cure to maintenance care was subtle. Two days later, Karen went on a 48-hour pass with her family. She returned from the pass very late one evening, and early the next morning, it was obvious that Karen was psychologically ready to die. She confirmed this by telling the team members that she was ready to die and needed to talk about it. This discussion threw all of the staff into somewhat of a panic. Although the staff were ready to begin to change from curing Karen to supporting her in the dying process, her rapid acceptance of her oncoming death and her overt expression of the desire to talk about it seemed to immobilize everyone.

In later discussions the staff concluded that there were probably several reasons for their shocked reaction; however, the two major ones were that (1) Karen assumed the role of leader in changing gears and inadvertently caused everyone else to experience real role conflict and (2) all the staff were emotionally attached to Karen and needed more time to successfully grieve.

Karen was approached by her primary nurse with the idea of having a psychiatrist join the team for the purposes of supporting the team (including Karen) as a whole in working through their feelings and providing Karen with someone to talk with who was ready to focus on *her* needs. (Other options, such as calling in a minister, were not chosen because of Karen's personal preferences.) The psychiatrist was able to provide considerable support to Karen and the other team members during that day and early evening. Karen went to

bed at 9:00 P.M. that evening and died at 4:45 A.M. the next morning. Her death occurred 96 days after her admission to the medical center.

At autopsy, Karen was found to have overwhelming cancer. Her lungs were more than half full of tumor. She also had metastasis throughout her body—in her brain, liver, gastrointestinal tract, spleen, pericardial sac and other organs.

REVIEW OF KAREN'S CARE

Looking back on the course of Karen's illness, one can say that she maintained her dignity and individuality as a person

---

Looking back on the course of Karen's illness, one can say that she maintained her dignity and individuality as a person throughout her illness.

---

throughout her illness. In working with Karen, the staff experienced firsthand some of the difficulties of trying to blend the cure model and the care model. Through the assignment of primary care givers, there was less confusion and increased continuity regarding goals of care.

Contracting served as a mechanism for making the goals, daily care activities and responsibilities of team members more explicit, as well as for meshing medical and nursing care plans. This also provided the patient with an explicit way of expressing needs and making priorities known. When the agreements of the contract are explicit, the patient has more control and independence. Implicit in this statement is the belief that a patient who has more control can achieve maximum functioning potential as a person.

Contracting offered a means of helping Karen function as a person. She had information available about her prognosis; people whom she trusted and knew would support her; control through an active role in determining her care; and probably decreased fear of the unknown. All of these points are important elements of the contracting approach, but the most important element of all was sharing—sharing information, control, joy and sorrow.

REFERENCES

1. Hammond, C.B. et al. "Treatment of Metastatic Trophoblastic Disease: Good and Poor Prognosis." *American Journal of Obstetrics and Gynecology* 115 (February 1973) p. 451–457.
2. *The American Heritage Dictionary of the English Language.* (Boston: Houghton Mifflin 1973) p. 289.
3. Zangari, M. and Duffy, P. "Contracting with Patients in Day-to-Day Practice." *American Journal of Nursing* 80:3 (1980) p. 451.
4. Steckel, S. "Contracting with Patient-Selected Reinforcers." *American Journal of Nursing* 80:9 (1980) p. 1596–1599.

The hospice movement: growing pains and promises

Patricia MacElveen-Hoehn, RN, PhD
Research Fellow
School of Nursing
University of Washington
Seattle, Washington

Elaine Graves McIntosh
Administrator
Hospice of Seattle
Seattle, Washington

SOCIAL MOVEMENTS arise out of dissatisfaction with the way things are and out of hopes for a better way. In the beginning the social movement lacks form or organization and relies on informal interactions with others with similar interests. Unconnected activities occur in different places; growth and development proceed at an uneven pace and often include reverses and setbacks. In informal discussions, the early innovators begin to formulate their ideas and to share them with others. Interest is generated, and more people become involved. Often the movement is nurtured by more general shifts in values that promote a climate within which the movement can continue to grow. Such a phenomenon is being witnessed today in the hospice movement. Many factors are contributing to its momentum, and growing experience with hospice efforts reveals many challenges that are internal to the delivery of this new approach.

0164-0534/81/0033-0029$2.00
© 1981 Aspen Systems Corporation

30

BIRTH OF THE HOSPICE CONCEPT

The humanitarianism of the 19th century provided the background for the gradual and pervasive shift of values that affected 20th century ideas about human rights and equality of opportunities in such areas as education, jobs and health. The traditional system of illness care in Western society has focused with great intensity and fervor on its struggles to diagnose and cure disease. Significant advances in knowledge and bio-technology increased the physician's ability to control and prolong life. Avoidance and inattention were common responses to dying persons who represented failure and defeat by the forces of nature. Some undesirable side effects of technological medicine became evident in the dehumanization of dying patients and the mechanical prolongation of their death.

During the 1960s several women began to pioneer the challenge of the patterns of care for the terminally ill. The first pioneer of the hospice movement was Cicely Saunders, with her background in medicine, nursing, social work and pharmacology. She founded St. Christopher's Hospice in London, which was dedicated to the care of the dying, research on pain and symptom management, and the design of a new approach to the more humane care for those patients and their families.[1]

Second was Jeanne Quint Benoliel, a nurse scientist, who through her research began articulating the problems in care for the dying that characterized the American care system. Of particular concern to her were the inadequate education and prepa-

ration of nurses to provide the kind of nursing care needed by terminally ill patients.[2] The third pioneer in the care of the dying was Elisabeth Kubler-Ross, a controversial psychiatrist who challenged physicians and others in the hospital system to listen to their dying patients and to learn from them. Her first book about dying and grief became a best seller in the popular press.[3] The next contributor was Florence S. Wald, who was dean of the Yale University School of Nursing when she first encountered Saunders. She then began a long series of efforts that later resulted in the establishment of the first American hospice at New Haven, Connecticut.[4]

St. Christopher's Hospice

Many American nurses involved in the care of terminally ill persons inspired by the hospice concept made pilgrimages to St. Christopher's to observe and learn.[5] The emphasis there was on care dependent on the use of caring people, with little or no emphasis on technology. The institution was rooted in a religious context and supported within the framework of a national health service system.

The approach to symptom control at St. Christopher's, especially pain management, was highly successful, and patients were kept mentally alert and comfortable, free of distress and free of the fear of pain. Once patients learned they could trust that comfort, they were able to use their energies for those activities that enriched the quality of their remaining life: knitting an afghan; visiting with their loved ones, including children and pets; enjoying their favorite music or being in the lovely gardens, where wheelchairs and beds were rolled out into the warm sunshine.

The patient was treated as a total person who had spiritual, emotional and social needs in addition to the needs for physical comfort. The patient and the family constituted the unit of care. The needs of family members as they anticipate a death and during their bereavement were part of the comprehensive model at St. Christopher's. The supportive, caring environment promoted for patients and families was extended to the professional staff and to the volunteers who were sharing the care.[6-11] Further, Saunders advised that the organizational structure of hospices be horizontal to allow administrators to be readily accessible to those receiving care, rather than the vertical hierarchy characteristic of the traditional medical care system.

Early phase of the hospice movement

Historically, a few established programs in this country provided excellent terminal care within the prevailing state of the art, but they remained isolated and external to the mainstream illness care system.[12] In contrast, the programs that developed within the hospice movement defined themselves as alternatives to the established system. The first of these programs, Hospice, Inc. (1971), grew out of the Interdisciplinary Study of Dying Patients and Their Families at Yale, with Florence Wald as the principal investigator. In Canada a few years later, Dr. Balfour Mount founded the Palliative Care Unit at Montreal's Royal Victoria Hospital.

In succeeding years of the 1970s, hospice programs developed at an increasingly rapid rate, with little or no connection with one another. This is typical of the behavior occurring in the early phase of a social reform movement, in which the initial activity is usually disorganized and in need of a leader who will give voice to the movement. In addition to the lack of a charismatic leader, the seeds of the hospice movement had been sown on secular soil.

In spite of these two seemingly major impediments, the new hospice groups continued to appear. In many places nurses familiar with the hospice concept tried to apply it within the limitations of their work settings. Many nurses extended their commitments to patients and families to provide consultation and support when they were not on duty and often voluntarily followed their clients who were discharged.

The hospice concept, with its respect for the needs of the whole person and the family members, was congruent with nursing's historic concern with total patient care, the growing concern for the members of the patient's social environment as a support system and the recognition of the family's own needs when a member was gravely ill. Thus the fit of nursing and hospice care was congruent and mutually supporting.

IDEOLOGY

Reform movements generally rally around values that have the essence of a basic good, and those attracted to the movement have a sense of mission.[13] In

32

English hospices, once pain and other symptoms were brought under control, it was possible for many patients to be at home. They were cared for by the family, who often could manage well with proper training, backup and support by the hospice staff. Most English hospices now offer a comprehensive program that includes in-hospice services for symptom management and respite care, home visits and day care.

In the day care program, patients may have a catheter changed and their hair washed and set. They probably will spend

---

It is said that the good death is to die in character, to have control over one's life so that there are no unwanted intrusions.

---

some time in the craft room working on a project and visiting with other patients and staff. It is a social occasion, time shared with friends, an outing to look forward to, and it also allows the primary caretaker at home to have a day off.

Generally, the hospice philosophy is characterized by the acceptance of death as a natural conclusion to life; hope can be offered so that patients will not feel isolated and abandoned. Their humanness and uniqueness are affirmed, and they have the right to live and die in a manner determined by them, rather than in a manner seen as ideal by the care providers.

The patient who has always been a fighter may want never to give up, thus choosing to die in that way. Occasionally, one sees the person who talks of what

bulbs to plant next spring or a journey that never will be made. It is said that the good death is to die in character, to have control over one's life so that there are no unwanted intrusions.

Distinguishing features of the hospice concept

Major aspects of hospice care that set it apart from most other terminal care can be outlined briefly as follows:

- *The patient and the family* together are considered the unit of care.
- *Comfort* is actively pursued through the control of physical, emotional, psychological and spiritual distress. More effective means for the management of most pain have been developed.
- An *interdisciplinary team* is involved in the planning and implementing of care. Patients and family members are considered integral members of the team.
- *Support is always available:* day or night, every day of the week.
- *Trained volunteers* are an essential component of any hospice program.
- *Bereavement* care and follow-up are provided for the family.
- *Support for care providers* is essential if staff and volunteers are willing to invest themselves if emotional exhaustion is to be averted.

There is considerable agreement that the bulk of hospice care currently being provided is nursing care, assistance with activities of daily living and household tasks. Nurses work directly with the patient's physician in the medical aspects of the patient's care needs. The expertise

Contrasting Case Examples

A lonely death

Upon the advice of the medical oncologist who had treated Mr. M's now metastatic disease for the past four years, he was admitted to a nursing home. The physician believed that the patient's care was too demanding for Mrs. M, who had some health problems of her own. Though she expressed willingness to take him home and considerable guilt over "deserting" her husband of 40 years, the physician and hospital personnel's influence and her fears about their concerns about her abilities caused Mrs. M to agree to the nursing home placement. The patient died three months later, having received twice weekly visits from his wife and one visit from his priest of many years. The couple's adult children and grandchildren had been encouraged not to visit the nursing home because it was "depressing."

A peaceful death at home

Mr. X, who had been diagnosed four years ago as having cancer of the lung, was returning home from the hospital following a course of palliative radiation. Though her husband's increasing disabilities and her own limitations due to arthritis created some fear in her competence to care for her husband, Mrs. X was reassured by the hospice nurse who visited her and her husband just prior to his discharge. The first three weeks at home were calm. In weekly visits the hospice nurse focused on maintaining Mr. X pain free, taught Mrs. X basic techniques for assisting her husband and encouraged the couple to reminisce about their long years together.

The social worker helped Mrs. X understand that her reluctance to learn the family finances was related to her fear and sadness at the impending loss of her husband. Gradually, she became increasingly able to discuss her feelings and finally allowed her husband to explain the details of their tax, insurance and financial status. Mr. X's knowledge that his wife was able to handle their affairs reassured him that she would "manage" after his death.

As the patient became increasingly ill, trusted friends from his church began bringing food and staying with him while Mrs. X slept or left the house for some time on her own.

Increasing and frequent pain caused the hospice nurse to suggest abandonment of the p.r.n. medication and initiation of the use of a pain cocktail on a scheduled basis around the clock. Children and grandchildren visited and assisted in the care of Mr. X. Family members were taught how to give injections of morphine, if needed, and gained comfort and confidence in the ability to share in his care.

The patient died peacefully one evening when the entire family was present.

---

of other professionals is utilized according to the specific issues confronting the patient and the patient's family. The team approach legitimizes the sharing of responsibilities. The combinations of team members who work with certain families are determined by the kinds of needs identified, the number of people being served and the assessment of their risks for problems prior to or following the patient's death.

A troublesome confusion in the tradi-

34

tional care system is that all care provided to patients is called "medical care." Components of hospice care also address other dimensions of care, for example, patients' and families' struggles with the meaning of life and of death, their review of important decisions made at an earlier time in life and their grief for lost opportunities or help to prepare children for a surrogate mother. The integration of trained volunteers who bring humanness, energy, skills and compassion adds yet another dimension to hospice care, which again is not "medical care."

The basic hospice philosophy has been translated into a variety of forms. Groups generated programs that were salient to their personal perspectives and the gaps in services they perceived in their communities. These forms are still emerging, although there are growing pressures to conform to the already defined models.

Models of hospice programs

Differences in the models of hospice programs are primarily a function of the settings in which they were launched. Some were independent of any parent institution or agency; others were affiliated with existing services.

The autonomous hospice in a free-standing building that offers inpatient care and services to the family is modeled after the English prototype. It may coordinate with existing home care programs in the community or expand its own services to include home care or day care.

The autonomous hospice home care program is totally involved with terminal care and does not provide home care to other kinds of patients. One type of program in this model provides skilled nursing within an interdisciplinary team approach. Another type does not offer "hands-on" nursing, but coordinates its supportive and counseling services with nursing from home health agencies through contractual or informal agreements. Another model is the lay volunteer program, which offers advocacy counseling and nonprofessional support to patients and their families.

Another approach to hospice care is the hospital-based program, which may have a defined unit for hospice beds. Another approach is the interdisciplinary hospice team, which provides consultation for terminally ill patients on all units in the hospital. In addition, many home health care agencies that have often cared for terminally ill patients are adding hospice care programs.

ORGANIZATION AND EXPANSION

Hospice groups continued to develop at a surprising rate. A sense of urgency promoted the formalization of a nationally visible group. Issues had emerged around the coordination of important efforts that would be required if the delivery of this innovation called hospice care would eventually qualify for reimbursement. By 1978 the National Hospice Organization held its first annual conference in Washington, D.C. and attracted more than a thousand people.

Some hospice groups received funding from state and federal agencies, foundation grants and public donations to start hospice demonstration programs. A few health care insurers entered into collaborative projects to study and evaluate hospice care.

During 1979 three significant statements were issued that articulated the scope and principles of care for the development of quality services for dying patients and their families. The first was the philosophical document published widely by the International Work Group on Death, Dying and Bereavement. This document proposed key assumptions and principles to provide guidelines for the development of standards for terminal care.[14] Concurrently, the American Nurses' Association Commission on Nursing Services adopted a compatible position with its approach of the Statement on Organized Care for the Terminally Ill and Their Families.[15]

Later that same year the Standards of a Hospice Program of Care developed by the National Hospice Organization (NHO) was distributed. These standards represented an effort to operationalize principles similar to those in the other two documents. This difficult challenge forced its writers to confront the traditional medical model, and in their sixth revision, these standards contain much emphasis on the roles of physicians and the medical care component.[16]

These important activities give testimony to the widespread recognition of the growth of the hospice movement and the proliferation of programs that were by their very nature on the periphery of the traditional care system. Because of their standing, they are not subject to regulation, nor eligible for third-party reimbursement.

Though many U.S. hospices have been successful in identifying "seed money" for one- to five-year demonstration projects,

the transition from initial funding to an ongoing, self-sustaining and stable financial basis is creating an environment ripe for organizational failures. Most hospices hope eventually to rely on third-party payers and patient fees for their "daily bread." At this time, however, reimbursement for full hospice care is a reality only in highly limited instances. Among these are persons eligible for Medicare and Medicaid being served by 26 organizations throughout the country, which are part of a special project in which the Health Care Financing Administration is paying for hospice care in order to determine costs and examine outcomes. Only after complete evaluation of this three-year study will efforts to amend current Medicare regulations be undertaken.

Simultaneous with this federal effort, some private insurance carriers are examining hospice care for effectiveness and reduction of health care costs associated with terminal care. Those within the hospice movement are faced with the challenge of proving that a true cost savings exists through the reduction of days of more costly hospital or other institutional care. In an era when the hue and cry over the high cost of health care resounds, leaders in the hospice movement must be successful in their efforts to demonstrate that cost savings are real and that hospice care will not simply be one more service that must be paid for.

CONFRONTATIONS AND CONFLICTS

The delivery of hospice care by those still close to its beginning ideology has

36   surfaced several philosophical and pragmatic issues at points where the innovative and the traditional conflict:

1. Respect for persons' rights to self-determination in how and when they want to live out the final stage of their lives is in contrast with the primacy of technology and its imposition. Though most existing patient bill of rights documents acknowledge the individual's right to decide, health care professionals accustomed to being in charge of patient care have great difficulty in both recognizing and changing the subtle ways they maintain control. Paternalism manifested by physicians and nurses in the giving of advice prior to exploring patient-family reactions, values and attitudes thwarts efforts to respect patient rights. Disapproval of certain patient decisions suggests the withdrawal of support and caring by the health care system and creates fear, which interferes with the client's confidence in the integrity of their choices.

2. The acknowledgement of the importance of spiritual and philosophical components of the phenomena of dying is tenuous. Will spiritual care be given lip service only or will time, energy and expertise—which can truly help people deal with spiritual issues and spiritual pain—be incorporated into the delivery of care?

3. Will the system accept the patient and family as the unit of care? What are the implications of this concept for the established patterns of providing and paying for care? Inclusion of family as legitimate recipients of service acknowledges that emotional care is properly placed in the domain of health care. The current system addresses the disease or the pathology, rather than the person as a social being with an illness. The hospice movement asks that the system expand to include not only total person needs, but also attention to nondiseased persons, the grieving family members.

4. Hospice supports the involvement of care providers with their clients. What are the risks to professionalism inherent in such involvement? Can providers learn how to sustain themselves through repeated loss of clients? Can a peaceful, anticipated and comfortable death become a worthy goal within the system and hence allow providers to feel a measure of satisfaction and success when it occurs? Given the approval for involvement, what are the obligations of agencies and institutions to lay and professional care providers? How is support for providers defined and institutionalized, and how is its cost absorbed?

5. Can the interdisciplinary team with truly shared leadership and responsibility become a functional reality? Can health care professionals accept others on the team, such as volunteers, counselors and clergy, as legitimate participants in the planning and provision of service? Will everyone defer to the physician in diffi-

cult situations, and will the physician allow this?

6. Will "the truth" be available to all patients, or will selection of patients "strong enough to be told" continue? Clearly, if the terminally ill are to be empowered to control their final months, they must know what is ahead for them biologically.

7. Will the ongoing need for research into new therapies impede the process of transferring control to the patient and family and yet respect their right to personal priorities over altruistic priorities?

8. Will the emphasis on efficiency and cost effectiveness in the evaluation of hospice-type care permanently obscure the quality of life values?

9. Will bereavement care be legitimized only if it can be proven to reduce immediate morbidity and mortality rates?

10. To what extent can hospice programs depend on the availability and commitment of unpaid volunteers as the excitement of a new approach yields to an established position?

11. How will the demand of standardization and accreditation influence the fate of those programs that emerge in response to local service needs rather than definitions of programs by external entities?

MODIFICATION AND COMPROMISE

As a social movement challenges the established patterns, the power of the status quo exerts enormous influence on the movement, especially as acceptance and legitimacy come closer to reality. The hospice movement has begun to have an impact on the system because it fills a painful gap. Success of the movement that could change the patterns of care for the terminally ill inside hospitals, nursing homes and home care programs would imply that special hospices or hospice programs were no longer necessary. An inherent danger exists in that as the system absorbs a new approach into itself, the pervasiveness of pressures to support the old and to avoid change can easily attenuate any impact.

Wald et al. caution strongly against premature standardization and incorporation of the reform that has not yet had its full opportunities to evolve and to explore its potential diversities.[17] However, as the idealists, who were the early starters of the movement, confront the constraints of the existing system, hard choices must be made. Which, if any, of the principles of hospice can be modified or abandoned and still maintain the integrity of the ideal? As seed monies become more scarce and competition for public and private support stiffens, will the energy and commitment to the movement survive through the struggles that lie ahead?

Hospice offers a unique opportunity to health care and social service providers. Within the hospice setting, holistic, sensitive and patient-centered care is possible.

Within the hospice setting, holistic, sensitive and patient-centered care is possible.

This is the type of environment that most providers were seeking when early career choices were made. If a united voice composed of consumers and providers can speak loudly to those who regulate and control the service delivery system, society may witness the birth of a whole new posture that holds great promise for those whose lives are touched by terminal illness.

REFERENCES

1. Benoliel, J.Q. *The Nurse and the Dying Patient* (New York: Macmillan 1967).
2. Saunders, C. "Care of the Dying." *Nursing Times Reprint* (London: Macmillan Publishers Ltd. 1963).
3. Kubler-Ross, E. *On Death and Dying* (New York: Macmillan 1969).
4. Wald, F. "Going Gently into that Good Night." *Mount Holyoke Alumnae Quarterly* 60:2(1976) p. 23.
5. Dobihal, S.V. "Hospice: Enabling a Patient to Die at Home." *American Journal of Nursing* 80 (August 1980) p. 1448-1451.
6. Saunders. "Care of the Dying."
7. Dobihal. "Hospice: Enabling a Patient to Die at Home."
8. Wald. "The Hospice Movement as a Health Care Reform." *Nursing Outlook* 28:3 (1980) p. 173-180.
9. McCorkle, R. "Hospices: A British Reality and an American Dream." (St. Louis: C.V. Mosby 1978) p. 125-131.
10. Plant, J. "Finding a Home for Hospice Care in the United States." *Hospitals, JAHA* 51 (July 1, 1977) p. 53-62.
11. Ingles, T. "St. Christopher's Hospice." *Nursing Outlook* 22:12 (1974) p. 759-763.
12. Wald. "The Hospice Movement as a Health Care Reform." p. 174.
13. Blumer, H. "Collective Behavior" in Lee, A.M., ed. *Principles of Sociology* (New York: Barnes and Noble 1967) p. 167-222.
14. International Work Group on Death, Dying and Bereavement. "Assumptions and Principles Underlying Standards for Terminal Care." *American Journal of Nursing* 79 (February 1979) p. 297-298.
15. American Nurses' Association Commission on Nursing Services. "Statement on Organized Care for the Terminally Ill and Their Families." (Approved February 10, 1979).
16. National Hospice Organization. *The Standards of a Hospice Program of Care*, 6th rev. (1979).
17. Wald. "The Hospice Movement as a Health Care Reform." p. 177.

A special Christmas:
an account of the last Christmas
of Barbara Mackenzie Rogers Hepner

Courtney Rogers Malone, MEd
Learning Disabilities Specialist
Public School System
Falmouth, Massachusetts

IT WAS GETTING-READY time—the week before Christmas when our three families were preparing to gather at our home near the sea in order to celebrate Christmas together in our usual fashion. As the house was decorated, presents wrapped, and food cooked, mixed feelings occupied our hearts and minds. We knew there would be a great deal of love. We hoped there would be some laughter and joy. We prayed there would be strength and courage, for this was to be my sister Bobby's last Christmas. She had been told by her doctor on December 17 that the cancer she had suffered had spread to her lungs. She would probably have two to three more months to live.

BOBBY'S FINAL WISH: DEATH WITH DIGNITY

Bobby was not particularly surprised by her doctor's prognosis for her, although she had felt well most of the fall. She had spent two years battling the physical

0164-0534/81/0033-0039$2.00
© 1981 Aspen Systems Corporation

40

demon as well as the mental ones. From time to time, she had experienced severe grief, anger and depression as well as long periods of serenity. But she also had been getting ready. By December 17, serenity had won over, and she asked us to help her to die as she had lived—with dignity and graciousness.

She told us that if it were possible, she would like to die at home. She signed a paper saying that she did not want life support systems to be used. She did not want to linger on, and she wanted to remain conscious if the pain could be kept within bearable bounds. Bobby prefaced each request with the statement that she did not want to burden anyone and would understand if some of her wishes could not be carried out.

There were two other wishes that I was asked to help fulfull. Dick, her husband, wanted to give her a warm bathrobe that would be lightweight and smooth next to her skin. Through my daughter in Boston, we found a perfect one which was filled with down. Bobby wanted to give Dick a fine gold watch, as he had never had one. She pulled her waning strength together for what had to be a very short outing. I fervently hoped there would be one she could afford in the village. We walked into the store, and there was just one. The perfect one. Bobby had it engraved to show their marriage dates: BRH–RHH, 1952–1980.

CHRISTMAS DAY

And so we gathered together. Bobby and Dick and their four grown children drove down from New Hampshire. Ray, her brother, and his wife Lois and their four children came from New Jersey. Al and I, with my children, welcomed them, and Christmas began.

Although we usually go to the midnight service together on Christmas Eve, Bobby was not strong enough to do so. Instead, on Christmas Day, we gathered in a circle in the living room to celebrate the Christmas Eucharist. Al, an Episcopal clergyman, led us in prayer, and Ray led us in song. In spite of the sorrow, we felt deeply thankful for the love our close-knit family had always shared. A great feeling of peace pervaded the house.

By Christmas night it was apparent that Bobby was weakening much more quickly than had been expected. We made her as comfortable as possible and propped her up on a myriad of pillows on a reclining chair to aid her breathing. She announced that she would stay there for the night, and Dick kept vigil on the couch.

It was as if Bobby had decided that now was the time, for she was with the people she loved most, and she was by the sea, which she loved. So she set about orchestrating her last days. Each day and through the nights we could see the life draining from her. Yet there were certain times when she willed herself to rally. On Christmas Day, we mustered up some of our usual jollity, and Bobby joined in the fun,

---

It was as if Bobby had decided that now was the time, for she was with the people she loved most, and she was by the sea, which she loved.

---

albeit from her chair of pillows. One could almost imagine that she might indeed have a few more months.

NEW YEAR'S EVE

By New Year's Eve, however, Bobby needed constant oxygen for two days and was exhausted by her efforts to breathe. Yet she wished to remain among us. Her sense of humor was still with her, as she smiled in appreciation of some of the jokes being told in the movie we were watching on television. However, she was determined to move on.

We asked for the help of a physician friend. Along with the oxygen machine, he supplied us with a painkilling medicine and the encouraging words that no one could do more for her than we were doing. He also offered us options that we could take if the nursing became too difficult for us: We could get the help of a homemaker or visiting nurse; he would arrange for a room at the local hospital, where we could be with Bobby as much as we wished; or we could have a hospital bed installed at home. He offered these options, but he did not insist on them. They were available if needed. We chose to order a bed and to nurse her ourselves. He also let us know where he would be at all times so that we could contact him personally if we needed him. We were very grateful for his support and understanding.

NEW YEAR'S DAY

By New Year's Day, Bobby's suffering was acute. We scheduled watches so that some could rest while others cared for her. But the watches went by the board, as no one would go to bed. Various members of the family, from a 16-year-old nephew on up, stayed by Bobby's side hour by hour. We felt that everything we did for her was a present so full of love that it was beyond measure. And yet they were all little things in themselves. We tenderly bathed her and fed her small spoonfuls of gelatin, which tasted refreshing to her. We held her hands and caressed her forehead. We played Chopin and Beethoven for her, and we cooled her lips with chunks of ice. We bought her the loveliest nightgown that could be found. We picked a green tiger lily leaf from our beloved summer home, "Lazy Lawn," and brought it to her. We sang carols around the piano and played duets on our recorders. Each in his or her own way told her and showed her what she meant to him or her and she in turn responded to each of us. It was a holy time.

That night Bobby's suffering became more acute. At the same time, her resolution grew firmer. As her lungs filled with fluid, she said, "Pray for courage."

We replied, "You have it."

Her response was, "I know it."

At 10:30, she tore off her oxygen mask and said, "Let's get on with it." She would not put it back on again.

Feeling the power of her spirit fighting to free itself from her body, we all gathered around her in the quiet light of the Christmas window candles. Al led us in prayers of thanks for her presence in our lives. He ended with, "Into thy hands, O merciful Saviour, we commend thy servant...." A daughter led us in singing "Amazing Grace." Each of us said good-

42

bye. Then Bobby looked at Dick, and as was her wont, whispered, "See you in the morning."

However, the battle was not yet won, and we continued to keep vigil throughout that long, still night. We were thankful for the beauty of the sky, with its brilliant stars and full moon, which augmented the candles. From time to time, we would step out onto the deck to catch a breath of fresh air and gather our thoughts. We found that we were still able to laugh a little when we discussed the evening meal, which Lois had named "God Knows Casserole." As the night waned, Bobby chose to take no more medicine. She was determined to remain lucid. And so she did. She was able to whisper an occasional word to us between her efforts to breathe.

BOBBY'S DEATH

The next afternoon, Bobby suddenly started breathing normally. She turned over on her side and arranged herself in her usual sleeping position. She opened her eyes wide and looked as if she was seeing something beyond us. Then she shut them and died. Although it was a very sad moment, we also felt triumphant. She was victorious, through sheer will and prayer, in living her last days as she had wished and in dying among us as she had hoped.

One of us proposed that we have a toast. I got out the best crystal goblets, and we filled them with sherry or ginger ale. We gathered around this dear person who had been our beloved wife, mother, sister and aunt. Then we raised our glasses as a son declared, "To Life!"

BOBBY'S FUNERAL

The funeral was a celebration. Bobby had planned it. Al and a family friend officiated. The simple pine casket was draped with our ancestral tartan with the family crest pinned to it. On top of this was a small bouquet of heather and mums from Dick. We sang the hymns lustily, and Ray played "Amazing Grace" on the bagpipes, because Bobby had asked him to. Al gave the sermon. Because it was the day before epiphany, he talked about gifts and reminded us that the Magi had had to go home another way after visiting the Christ child. It was fitting, because we realized that not only had Bobby's presence among us over the years been a gift beyond measure, but the intangible gifts we had all been giving and receiving during that Christmas season were mighty treasures. Because we would no longer have Bobby among us, and because of our experiences, we all knew that life would be different, and we indeed would be going home another way.

BOBBY'S VICTORY: ALLOWING THE TERMINALLY ILL TO DIE AT HOME

I have written this account in hopes that the experience of our family may be of some help to others. As death after long

---

We discovered inner strength we were not sure we had by committing ourselves to Bobby's wish to die at home.

illness has become so common in our modern age, we all wonder before the fact how best to deal with it. Medicine can do much, but the time comes when life and death, and the quality of them, transcend science. This can be a fearful realization, but it can also be a glorious one. Not every family can manage death, or might want to, as we did. We were given several options by our physician friend. There is also the hospice movement, which is devoted to enabling the terminally ill to live more fully their last days. We discovered inner strength we were not sure we had by committing ourselves to Bobby's wish to die at home. We are all very glad we did. We thank her for teaching us so much about life as she let go of hers.

The impact of sudden infant death on the family: nursing intervention

Sally Nikolaisen, R.N., M.N.
Assistant Professor of Nursing
Seattle Pacific University
Seattle, Washington

DEATH, whether sudden or expected, leaves in its path a family in distress. The sudden, unexpected death of a loved one is a tragic experience, and in our death-denying society, few families are prepared to handle the loss of a member.

The loss of a loved one influences multiple areas of individual and family functioning: social, physical, and psychological. Families that experience the death of a family member are at high risk for developing illnesses or other complications. An increase in mortality and morbidity in survivors during the first six months following the death of a loved one has been reported. The sudden, unexpected death of a loved one is thought to have the most profound effects on survivors.[1-5]

SUDDEN INFANT DEATH SYNDROME

Sudden death is no respecter of age or family condition. Accidents cause the greatest number of deaths among children,

0164-0534/81/0033-0045$2.00

46

adolescents and young adults, whereas cardiovascular diseases are responsible for more deaths among adults.[6] The cause of death that is perhaps the most difficult to understand and cope with is Sudden Infant Death Syndrome (SIDS). There is no way of predicting this disease, no method of prevention and no way to reverse its effects. Sudden Infant Death Syndrome claims the lives of more infants under one year of age than any other known cause.[7]

Because of its suddeness, the death of an infant catches parents unprepared to deal with an overwhelming situation. The sudden loss of an apparently healthy infant can have devastating effects on each person in the family as well as the family as a unit. Parents who are victims of unexplained or misdiagnosed deaths of their children often report feelings of despondency and inadequacy. In an attempt to find a reason for the death, they often blame themselves or their spouses for having failed in some way. The parents' perception of the loss is further distorted and complicated by their acute grief response.[8,9]

PARENTS' RESPONSES TO THE SUDDEN DEATH OF THEIR INFANT

Parents who lose a child to SIDS often report grief responses similar to the responses described by Lindemann in his classic study of grief responses of the survivors of the tragic Coconut Grove fire.[10] In the acute phase, disbelief and shock are the initial responses, followed by reality testing.

Many parents speak of the infant in a combination of present and past tenses. Mothers in particular may be disturbed by the fact that they think they hear the infant crying and go to the nursery, or they prepare for the infant's bath or make formula before they realize what they are doing. These reactions may last several weeks. Parents also describe feelings of anger, helplessness and loss of meaning in life and may be fearful, especially for their surviving children. Guilt feelings are universal and pervasive.[11-14]

Physical and emotional responses

The physical symptoms of grief are often alarming to parents. Parents complain of strange visceral sensations, such as "whirling around," "pressure in the head," "heartache" and "stomach pains." They describe feeling lumps in the throat and a choking sensation, and their appetite and sleep habits are frequently disrupted.

Parents' emotional symptoms of grief are reflected in their affect: they often appear depressed and exhibit slow movements, sighing, insomnia, restlessness or excessive activity. Depression is a normal component of grief and should not be interpreted as undesirable.[15-17]

Psychological effects and effects on familial relationships

Many parents who experience the loss of an infant are young couples just beginning the process of developing their relationship with each other. Young people in American society generally have had little, if any, experience with death. Thus the sudden, unexpected death of their infant has a profound impact on young couples' relationships.[18] They frequently are just beginning to adjust to being a family unit at the time of their loss.

Most infants die of SIDS at the age when they are beginning to respond to others in a social way with smiles and coos. Since mothers have generally had the primary care for the infant, the sudden loss can be particularly devastating for them.

Mothers whose infants die of SIDS often experience wide mood swings and difficulty concentrating, and they frequently express hostile feelings toward even their closest friends and relatives.

Mothers whose infants die of SIDS often experience wide mood swings and difficulty concentrating, and they frequently express hostile feelings toward even their closest relatives.

They report feeling ambivalent toward surviving children. At times they are fearful for them and want to overprotect them; at other times they become impatient with them and more easily irritated and upset by their behavior.[19,20]

The mother may want desperately to talk about her pain and the infant, but her partner may not be receptive. He may not be able to tolerate her pain or may rationalize that if she stops talking about the infant, the pain will cease.

Parents often do not know how to talk with each other about the severe stress of their loss, and communication often breaks down. They may try to protect one another by hiding their feelings. Although they hide their real fears, concerns and anxieties from each other, their behaviors are observable, and the major differences in their grieving responses serve to widen the gap between them.[21,22]

A father who has suffered the death of an infant may appear to lose himself in his work and may act as if the death did not bother him, which may give others the impression that he really did not care about the infant. Many of the differences between the responses of fathers and mothers to losing a child are created by societal role expectations that men are tough and protective and do not cry or show emotional feelings. As a result, fathers often are left out or isolate themselves from the family grieving process. Some fathers may feel the need to flee from their spouses' grieving behavior by becoming immersed in work or in other activities that keep them away from home.[23]

In Lindemann's study, it was the seemingly courageous people who in time were defeated by death. Months or perhaps years later, they developed definite signs of mental illness.[24] Couples often report feeling as though they are behaving inappropriately because they are grieving when those around them seem to be doing well. Friends and relatives may be perceived to be in a conspiracy of silence concerning the death in order to protect the parents.[25]

Parents frequently are unable to face the needs of the surviving siblings unless urged to do so. Their inability to face the needs of their children is probably related to several factors:

- the desire to protect them from the pain and reality of death;
- the lack of awareness that children can

understand death and do grieve, although their behaviors may differ from those of adults;

- a preexistent communication gap between parent and child; and
- the parents' preoccupation with their own grief and pain.[26]

CHILDREN'S RESPONSES TO THE LOSS OF A SIBLING

Children are particularly vulnerable to the effects of a major loss suffered early in life. Their responses are sometimes obvious immediately, or they may emerge many decades later. The most disturbing effect on the children of a family crisis is the inability of significant adults to provide ego support and control. Adults who are caught in the emotional web of their own grief may not be able to recognize or respond to the needs of their children.[27,28]

Effects of changing roles in the family

The practice of preparing children for the birth of a new sibling makes them a part of this significant event in the family history. The birth of an infant becomes an organizing factor around which new roles of all family members are crystallized. When the role of older sibling is interrupted by the death of an infant, the surviving sibling must deal with the absence of the new member of the family. The surviving sibling is intellectually and emotionally poorly equipped to resolve the loss. The child experiences not only the loss of the sibling but also the grief of the parents and probably some changes in his or her relationship with them.[29,30]

Effects of parents' attitudes toward and reactions to death

Adults' attitudes toward death are sensed by children. When the parents are overwhelmed by the death of an infant and are unable to come to grips with their own feelings, the surviving children absorb their anxiety. If the parents are afraid to talk about the death, the children may remain silent and repress fears and feelings of guilt and confusion.[31]

The surviving children are sensitive to the parents' mood and behavior changes, as the parents progress through the phases of bereavement: the shock and denial of the loss, the developing awareness of the loss and the work of mourning. Cain found that in at least one-fourth of the children experiencing loss, the primary impact of the sibling's death consisted of the parents' profound grief reactions and prolonged mourning.

In the initial phase of grief, parents have little energy to devote to their surviving children. The parents no longer respond in a previously predictable fashion. As they move through the grief process, they communicate a lability of mood that can be very frightening to the children. When this occurs, children see the foundation of their security wavering, and they feel threatened. Mothers may sometimes act withdrawn, preoccupied and depressed; at other times, they may act overprotective and smothering. Children are often confused by these contradictory behaviors. Fathers may often seem calm and stoic and appear to function effectively, but often they hear little of what is said to them, constantly forget things, become muted and display automatonlike behavior.[32]

Grieving parents can be helped to understand their own reactions during the bereavement period and what their children may be experiencing. Children are most effectively helped to cope with the death of a sibling by their parents, and they tend to be resilient if they have the security and strength of family togetherness. Parents in turn need help in providing support to their children at a time when their own coping energy is at a low ebb.

THE ROLE OF THE COMMUNITY HEALTH NURSE IN GRIEF COUNSELING

Nurses are especially qualified to counsel grieving families. They are prepared to handle the medical questions raised by families and to provide grief counseling and support. During the initial phase of shock, the nurse may see the family in the hospital emergency room, where the family members need to be assisted in coping with their grief. At this point, families can be supported by the presence of a nurse who is sensitive to their pain and confusion. The nurse can offer practical help in arranging for social services to assist with details, such as funeral arrangements and child care.

Community health nurses are ideally suited to provide information and counseling to grieving parents after they leave the hospital. Community health nurses, by virtue of their education and experience, have performed credibly in the dual role of explaining medical information and providing grief counseling.

A community health nurse has a basic knowledge of the physical aspects of SIDS and of basic grief responses. A community health nurse educated for SIDS counseling is generally comfortable discussing physiological problems with families and is able to give adequate interpretations of the pathological findings and answer parents' questions regarding the death in an informed and confident manner.

The prepared community health nurse is also knowledgeable about basic grief responses and thus is able to respond to the parents' needs. Nurses who work with families that have recently lost a child often seek consultation themselves from a qualified mental health professional. Such counseling provides the nurses with the opportunity to work through their feelings regarding the grieving families' problems, as well as the nurses' personal experiences with loss and grief, which can be restimulated and limit their objectivity.[33]

The SIDS program

In 1969 a research team at Children's Orthopedic Hospital in Seattle, Washington interviewed SIDS parents to gather epidemiological information. The nurse who conducted the interviews found that in the process of gathering information, she was providing parents with information about SIDS and counseling regarding the grief process. When the research was completed, it was recommended that this service be continued.[34,35]

Based on this research, the Seattle King County Health Department, in cooperation with Children's Orthopedic Hospital, developed a program for SIDS counseling. The program, which has been cited as a model for grief counseling, stresses four major points:

1. prompt identification of SIDS as a preliminary cause of death (within 24 to 48 hours) by means of autopsy or other acceptable standards;
2. use of correct diagnostic terminology, that is, SIDS, on the death certificate;
3. notification of the family as soon as identification of SIDS has been established; and
4. provision of facts regarding SIDS and of grief counseling by a specially prepared public health nurse.

Nurses in King County alone visit 50 to 60 families yearly.[36]

Home visits for grief counseling

It is generally recognized that it takes one to two years for families to regain the level of personal happiness felt before the death of a loved one. The focus of counseling grieving families is preventive mental health and family advocacy. Various time frames have been recommended for counseling visits to grieving families.[37-39] The following are broad guidelines for making grief counseling visits based on the extensive experience of the Seattle King County Health Department.

The initial visit: assessing the needs of the family

Nurses are responsible for assessing the unique needs of each family. The first visit is usually made within the first two weeks following the death. At this time, families are often concerned about the reason for their infant's death. The nurse provides as much factual information relating to the cause of death as possible, in simple terminology.

Because they are flooded with feelings of anger and disbelief, families often are unable to hear or understand detailed explanations. One of the most important behaviors for the nurse during this visit is listening, with the goal of finding out what is really bothering the family and its individual members.[40]

Providing emotional support

Nurses can effectively assist families in expressing their feelings by realizing the importance of being with the family as a caring human being. The greatest need of grieving families is to have someone who is objective and genuinely interested.

Frequently, just being given permission to feel anger decreases parents' feelings of guilt about the death of their infant.

Nurses should be careful to avoid projecting their own feelings about what the family should be experiencing on the family and should instead try to assess what the family members are actually feeling.[41]

Nurses give grieving parents assurance that they will not always feel the intense pain of this moment, that grieving takes time and that only time will make the difference. It is helpful for nurses to share with families that many parents experience a sense of helplessness and resultant anger at not having been able to prevent their infant's death. The nurse should let them know that there is reason to feel anger and that it is OK. Frequently, just being given permission to feel anger decreases parents' feelings of guilt about the death of their infant.[42]

Normalizing the grief process

One of the major focuses of the early counseling sessions is to normalize the grief process. Families are helped to understand that the grief process is universal and a common experience of families who have lost infants to SIDS.

Use of the third person is often effective in helping parents identify feelings that can be frightening. An example of this is to share with parents, "It is often reported by parents that they hear their infant cry or find themselves getting the infant's bottle ready. Has anything like this happened to you?" Frequently, parents will say they have had similar experiences. The nurse can then assure them that this is normal. The sense of relief that this knowledge brings to parents is often visible in a change in their affect.[43]

Grief is a personal feeling, and persons in the same family can differ greatly in their grief reactions. It is helpful for a couple to know that there frequently are differences between male and female expressions of grief. By opening the lines of communication between the mother and father, the nurse encourages the parents to provide needed support to each other. The nurse also reinforces the strengths and assets of each partner and of the family as a group.[44]

Assessing physical effects on the family

The community health nurse assesses the physical responses of the family, especially the mother. A mother may have been breastfeeding her infant at the time of the infant's death and therefore may have been left with physical pain and discomfort in addition to mental anguish. The nurse also assesses the eating and sleeping patterns of the family and offers suggestions for ensuring proper diet and rest.

Helping the children

It is important for the community health nurse to be aware of the needs of surviving siblings and to help the parents to do likewise. Emphasis is placed on helping the parents help the siblings, and parents may be encouraged to have the children present for some of the home visits.

Once rapport is established with the children, the nurse can ask about the children's beliefs regarding the infant's death and related concerns. Misconceptions and fantasies that may be causing problems can then be clarified. If the child feels threatened or is too young to verbalize concerns directly, the nurse can give the child emotional support indirectly: "Sometimes sisters and brothers don't like new babies and feel they are a real pain. The baby's death had nothing to do with these feelings. Feelings don't cause someone to die."[45]

Scheduling visits

The time span between the first home visit to a grieving family and follow-up visits and the frequency of home visits will depend on the unique needs of the family and the resources of the community health agency. It is recommended that a second visit be made during the first six weeks and another within the next three months. Follow-up visits around one year after the infant's death are also important. The family may have a difficult time on the child's birthday, major holidays and the anniversary of the death. Home or phone

52

visits on these dates would be most help-ful.

The family is given the nurse's name and telephone number and is encouraged to call whenever the need arises. Families often report that just knowing there is someone they can call if needed helps them through rough times.

At the time of follow-up visits, the nurse may perceive that a family is in need of more intensive help in coping with the loss. Families that have a history of emotional instability, that have experienced another recent death or that have a previous unresolved loss may be especially vulnerable. Individuals who have a history of mental illness are also at high risk.

Families that seem to be exhibiting a complete disruption in communication or that seem headed for a break-up may need family therapy. Individuals who show signs of a prolonged, exaggerated or delayed grief reaction, symptoms of depressive illness, severe psychosomatic illness or severe behavioral problems may need the help of a professional mental health worker.

It is impossible to predict in the first few months following their loss which families will successfully work through their grief. It is recommended that intervention with families that have experienced a sudden death be continued for a minimum of two years. The value of immediate professional intervention for these families is recognized. However, when this support is not available initially, later intervention by community health nurses can help to facilitate healthy family adaptations.[46]

THE GROWTH OF SIDS PROGRAMS

A great deal of progress has been made since 1970, when six community health nurses in King County, Washington provided assistance to families who had lost infants to SIDS. As of October 1980 37 states (including the District of Columbia) have developed SIDS projects that identify cases of SIDS and provide information and counseling services for the survivors. Legislation has been passed that requires each state, territory and possession to have a SIDS project by the end of 1981.[47]

Many advances have been made toward identifying possible causes of SIDS, and indications are that there are multiple causes. However, it is still not possible to clearly identify infants at risk prior to death. The destructive effects of SIDS go far beyond the lost lives of infants; the suffering of surviving family members can be devastating.

Reactions to death will vary according to the social, emotional and spiritual resources of the individuals involved. Support and skilled counseling from a community health nurse at critical points can help families dispel guilt, calm fears, restore relationships, rebuild confidence and reestablish stable and healthy functioning.[48]

REFERENCES

1. Kubler-Ross, E. *Questions and Answers on Death and Dying.* (New York: Macmillan 1974) p. 60–68.
2. Defrain, J.D. and Ernst, L. "The Psychological Effects of Sudden Infant Death Syndrome on Surviving Family Members." *The Journal of Family Practice* 6:2 (1978) p. 985–989.

3. Secundy, M.G. "Bereavement: The Role of the Family Physician." *Journal of the National Medical Association* 69:9 (1977) p. 650.

4. Kubler-Ross. *Questions and Answers on Death and Dying.* p. 60-68.

5. Defrain and Ernst. "The Psychological Effects of Sudden Infant Death Syndrome." p. 985-989.

6. National Safety Council. *Accident Facts.* (Chicago: NSC 1978) p. 8-9.

7. Beckwith, J.B. *The Sudden Infant Death Syndrome* DHEW Pub. No. (HSA) 75-5137 (Washington, D.C.: Government Printing Office 1975).

8. Ibid.

9. Stitt, A. "Emergency after Death." *Emergency Medicine* Reprint (March 1971) p. 270-279.

10. Lindemann, E. "Symptomatology and Management of Acute Grief." *American Journal of Psychiatry* 101 (September 1944) p. 141-148.

11. Stitt. "Emergency after Death." p. 270, 271.

12. Patterson, K. and Pomeroy, M.R. "Nursing Care Begins after Death When the Disease is Sudden Infant Death Syndrome." *Nursing '74* 4 (May 1974) p. 85-88.

13. Smialek, Z. "Observations on Immediate Reactions of Families to Sudden Infant Death." *Pediatrics* 62 (January 1978) p. 160-165.

14. Secundy. "Bereavement: The Role of the Family Physician." p. 650.

15. Bergman, A.B. "Sudden Infant Death Syndrome: An Approach to Management." *Primary Care* 3 (March 1976) p. 1-8.

16. Miles, M.S., ed. *The Mental Health Aspects of Sudden Infant Death Syndrome (SIDS).* Report of a conference sponsored by the National Foundation for Sudden Infant Death and the National Institute of Mental Health, Kansas City, Missouri, July 30, 1975 (New York: National Foundation for Sudden Infant Death, 1975).

17. Defrain and Ernst. "The Psychological Effects of Sudden Infant Death Syndrome." p. 985-989.

18. Nikolaisen, S.M. and Williams, R.A. "Parents' View of Support Following the Loss of Their Infant to Sudden Infant Death Syndrome." *Western Journal of Nursing Research* 2:3 (1980) p. 594.

19. Szybist, C. *The Subsequent Child.* (New York: National Sudden Infant Death Syndrome Foundation, 1976).

20. Miles. *The Mental Health Aspects of Sudden Infant Death Syndrome (SIDS).* p. 2.

21. Nikolaisen and Williams. "Parents' View of Support Following the Loss of Their Infant." p. 594.

22. Smialek. "Observations on Immediate Reactions of Families." p. 160-165.

23. Patterson and Pomeroy. "Nursing Care Begins after Death." p. 85-88.

24. Lindemann, "Symptomatology and Management of Acute Grief." p. 141-148.

25. Helmrath, T.A. and Steinitz, E.M. "Death of an Infant: Parental Grieving and the Failure of Social Support." *The Journal of Family Practice* 6:4 (1978) p. 785-790.

26. Stitt, "Emergency after Death." p. 270-279.

27. Cain, A.C. et al. "Children's Disturbed Reactions to the Death of a Sibling." *Journal of Orthopsychiatry* 34:4 (1964) p. 741-753.

28. Moriarity, D.M., ed. *The Loss of Loved Ones: The Effects of Death in the Family on Personality Development* (Springfield, Ill.: Charles C Thomas 1967).

29. Hardgrove, C. and Warrick, L.H. "How Shall We Tell the Children?" *American Journal of Nursing* 74:3 (1974) p. 448-450.

30. Hagan, J. "Nursing Interaction and Intervention with Grieving Families" in *After Our Baby Died: Instructor's Guide for a film on the Sudden Infant Death Syndrome* DHEW Pub. No. (HSA) 76-5141 (Washington, D.C.: Government Printing Office 1976) p. 7-13.

31. Hardgrove and Warrick. "How Shall We Tell the Children?" p. 448-450.

32. Ibid.

33. Miles. *The Mental Health Aspects of Sudden Infant Death Syndrome (SIDS).* p. 1.

34. Patterson and Pomeroy. "Nursing Care Begins after Death." p. 85.

35. Bergman. "Sudden Infant Death Syndrome." p. 1-8.

36. Nikolaisen and Williams. "Parents' View of Support Following the Loss." p. 595.

37. Defrain and Ernst. "The Psychological Effects of Sudden Infant Death Syndrome." p. 985-989.

38. Helmrath and Steinitz. "Death of an Infant." p. 785-790.

39. Miles. *The Mental Health Aspects of Sudden Infant Death Syndrome (SIDS).* p. 3-11.

40. Ibid.

41. Hagan. "Nursing Interaction and Intervention with Grieving Families." p. 7-13.

42. Smialek. "Observations on Immediate Reactions of Families." p. 160-165.

43. Hagan, J. "Nursing Interaction and Intervention with Grieving Families." p. 7-13.

44. Helmrath and Steinitz. "Death of an Infant." p. 785-790.

45. Miles. *The Mental Health Aspects of Sudden Infant Death Syndrome (SIDS).* p. 6.

46. "Special Report: Nurse's Grief Intervention Two Years after SIDS Death Saves Family." *Thanatology Today* 2:9 (1980) p. 3-4.

47. Ibid.

48. Limerick, L. "Cot-Deaths: The Bereaved Parents' Need for Support." *Midwives Chronicle and Nursing Notes* 90 (October 1977) p. 231-234.

The patient's need of faith at death

R. Larry Shelton, ThD
Director of the School of Religion
Seattle Pacific University
Seattle, Washington

THE REALITY of impending death brings home the need for persons to enlist coping systems that have adequately sustained them in previous times of crisis. Since people tend to be more responsive in crises to those systems that have proven adequate in the past, it is important that patients who subscribe to religious faith be encouraged to utilize this faith to cope with the vulnerability and fear of death. A number of aspects of faith can provide patients with a sense of spiritual adequacy and serenity in the terminal crisis.

FAITH AND HUMAN EXISTENCE

At no time do the basic questions of human existence assert themselves more insistently than at death. The patient may ponder why death comes now. What is the nature of life after death? What does death mean? Answers need to be found that bring meaning, peace and strength to the dying.

0164-0534/81/0033-0055$2.00
© 1981 Aspen Systems Corporation

56

Faith provides a cultural context

In every culture, attempts are made to explain the meaning of existence, and these cultural expressions bring comfort to the dying. Various representations of death in animistic cultures reflect the vividness with which life after death is imagined. The various representations of life after death as a beautiful land in some of the Oriental religions reflect the attempts of these cultures to find meaning. The Christian conception of eternal life involving interpersonal communion with God enables the patient to gain meaning by identifying with the hope within this tradition.

Trelease relates the poignant saga of Old Sarah, an Alaskan matriarch who prepared carefully for her death. She summoned the priest to come on a certain day and also gathered together all the members of her family. In the morning of the appointed day, she had planned a time of prayer for each member of her family, then a great celebration of the Eucharist in her cabin in a service that included numerous hymns and prayers. She participated joyfully and seemed very content and fulfilled. After the worship activities were completed, everyone left, and she died shortly afterward.[1]

Old Sarah found peace and meaning in the faith that had served her well for many years, and the Alaskan Indian cultural understanding of her responsibility to others at her time of death formed the folkway that was enacted in the closing ceremonies of her life.

Faith helps find answers

In the teaching and experience of faith, answers to the ultimate questions of life and death are found. Satisfactory systems of belief bring a sense of resolution and peace to the terminally ill patients who find in this faith meaningful truth and hope. This hopeful acceptance of death and life after death brings creativity and comfort to the experience of dying. The debilitating fear of the unknown is overcome by confident trust in the answers of faith.

Spiritual insights are gained and values are developed and clarified by the understanding that death is not only catastrophic and destructive, but can be the motivation for creative growth.[2] The spiritual resources and literature of religious faith enable a person to explore the issues of life after death, the meaning of pain and personal ethical responsibility. Not only are the answers to these ultimate questions sources of strength for the individual, but the process of questioning itself opens the person to various facets of truth and the meaning of spiritual discovery.

FAITH AND TRANSITION

Faith provides a rationale for transition

"Dying should be seen as a phase of living and subject to growth and obligations and opportunities just as is every other phase of living."[3] Personality continues to develop, and faith provides definition, values and motivation for

---

A faith that provides adequately for an explanation of life beyond death enables the patient to place death within a manageable perspective.

growth. When the self is perceived as being too valuable for extinction, death is understood not as the end, but as the transition from one aspect of human existence to another.[4] In the context of faith, the patient overcomes fear of death and sees it as both the completion of life and the transition to a new life.[5] A faith that provides adequately for an explanation of life beyond death enables the patient to place death within a manageable perspective. It ceases to be an ogre and becomes a natural stage in the development of human existence.

Faith provides an agenda for growth

When death is faced realistically and with the hope of life after death, it can provide an enriching perspective on the meaning and purposes of life. Faith can be the foundation for purpose even when the possibilities of extended life expectancy vanish. Faith can contribute an agenda for growth as the patient puts affairs in order and responds to opportunities for growth in understanding, love and hope.

This growth of the spirit in the face of physical deterioration can be seen in the case of Woody, a man who contracted lateral sclerosis; his story is told effectively in an account by his wife.[6] In a tremendously courageous pilgrimage of faith, Woody amazed those around him with his tender and increasingly feeble expressions of love for God and his family and his effective and often poignant attempts to bring others to maturity and faith. He learned to see the beauty of flowers and snowflakes and developed a personal faith, spiritual maturity and family intimacy that crowned the conclusion of his life with fulfillment.

A part of final growth in preparation for death is the integration of the death experience into all of life. In the context of faith, death can be seen as the completion of a life well lived, a fulfillment of a lifetime of development. It can be understood as the beginning of the realization of all the hopes and expectations of life after death. Faith enables persons to place their dependency in divine wisdom, and to avoid succumbing to bitterness and frustration, and thus to find confidence as life ebbs.

Faith provides a support system

An important value of life is the sense of relationship to those who have shared the victories and defeats of life in the past. The security found in identification with a reference point more permanent than the self significantly enhances and heals the spirit. The Egyptian and American Indian burial rituals involved equipping the deceased with implements necessary to function in the afterlife and indicated faith in being united with those who had lived before.

Christian worship, as understood within the Roman Catholic, Orthodox and Protestant traditions, provides rituals that bring unity and identity with Jesus and a tradition of faith and fellowship with others across the ages. Other religions have identifying rituals that help their members understand and express faith in some higher power. Participation in these rituals gives identification with the past and hope for the future while enriching both the conscious and preconscious mind with their symbolism.[7]

The participation in the symbolic drama of rituals of faith fulfills mental and

58

emotional needs by involving the participant in the larger cosmic drama that forms the foundations for faith. The symbolic reliving of the events of Jesus' passion prepares Christian patients for death by enabling them to incorporate the elements of life and death into their own experiences and to identify with the life and death of one who overcame death because of his submission to God. Furthermore, in the absolution of the Lord's Supper, the patient can be relieved of guilt, real or neurotic, can move away from preoccupation with the past and can anticipate the newness of life in the future.[8]

In Judaism death is not the end of life, but the end of physical existence. Life created by God continues through one's descendants and personal influence as well as through the immortality of the soul, which is indestructible.[9] The practice of confession, in which forgiveness is sought with the prayer, "May my death be an atonement for all my sins," reflects a desire for purification of sins through death. A request for God's love and mercy and a petition to be transported after death into a life with God follow, and the Shema, which Jewish believers have recited twice a day for their entire lives, is repeated: "Hear, O Israel, the Lord our God is one Lord. . . ." (Deuteronomy 6:4). With this familiar ritual, the Jewish person feels prepared for death and is released to enjoy immortality and a reunion with God.[10]

FAITH AND PROFESSIONAL HEALTH CARE

The health care professional can assist greatly in bringing peace and integration to the dying by being able to appreciate and understand the spiritual needs of the patient. This holistic concern can provide the terminally ill with critically needed resources as they face the fear and strangeness of death and the unfamiliarity of their surroundings.

Faith of the patient provides a point of entry for support

The professional may find it difficult to find an entry point for support for terminally ill patients, particularly if they have not resolved the issue of acceptance of death or if they are depressed and confused. Patients who have a functioning faith may be approached supportively from the perspective of their belief system. Affirmation of the patient's dependence on a system of faith opens up potential channels of communication and strengthens the capacity to cope with the stress of dying.

While discussion of domestic or other personal topics may become unsettling to the dying, encouraging patients to elaborate on the emotional and spiritual aspects of their faith enhances their growth and personality integration. It is important, however, that these conversations not be judgmental or controversial. If patients feel accepted and affirmed in their religious beliefs, the possibility of their opening up other, perhaps more intimate, areas of concern is increased.

Faith of the professional makes possible a relationship of empathy

If the professional shares a system of faith similar to that of the patient, a very important support relationship may develop. Even when the patient and the professional are of different faiths, an attempt to understand the patient's ultimate concerns is crucial. The ability to share honestly, intelligently and supportively with patients about the implications of their faith makes an empathic approach to their needs possible. It is through such a relationship of caring support that the most effective holistic health care is accomplished.

REFERENCES

1. Trelease, M. "Dying among Alaskan Indians: A Matter of Choice" in Kubler-Ross, E., ed. *Death: The Final Stage of Growth* (Englewood Cliffs, N.J.: Prentice-Hall 1975) p. 34–35.
2. Kubler-Ross, E., ed. *Death: The Final Stage of Growth* (Englewood Cliffs, N.J.: Prentice-Hall 1975) p. 1–3.
3. Trealease. "Dying among Alaskan Indians." p. 36.
4. Heller, Rabbi Z. "The Jewish View of Death: Guidelines for Dying" in Kubler-Ross. *Death: The Final Stage of Growth.* p. 38.
5. Winter, D. *Hereafter: What Happens after Death?* (Wheaton, Ill.: Harold Shaw 1972) p. 13.
6. Shelton, B. and Terrell, B. *Woody* (Chappaqua, Ill: Christian Herald Publications 1979).
7. Jackson, E. *Understanding Grief* (New York: Abingdon 1957) p. 117, 124.
8. *Ibid.* p. 127, 128.
9. Levine, R. H. *Holy Mountain: Two Paths to One God* (Portland: Binfords and Mort 1953) p. 39.
10. Conversation with Rabbi James L. Mirel, PhD, Temple De Hirsch Sinai, Seattle, Washington, March 5, 1981.

Near-death events and critical care nursing

Annalee R. Oakes, RN, MA, CCRN
Associate Professor and Instructor of
Emergency-Care Nursing
Seattle Pacific University
Seattle, Washington

A FEW WEEKS before Mr. Edward C. died of cancer, he visited a close friend who was also dying of cancer. It was obvious to any observer that his friend was wasted and pitifully weak, very near death, yet extremely anxious to discuss a pressing concern. In low tones, the dying man whispered this question: "Ed, do you think there is any life after death?"

People through the ages have pondered that same question and have reflected wonderment about the answer by living and dying in a variety of ritualistic ways. (See "Societal/Cultural Views Regarding Death and Dying," by H. M. Ross in this issue.) Until recently most people who died were not revived. Isolated incidents of people supposedly dead but somehow revived were considered miracles, and any associated reports by the victims or their families took on mythical connotations. Consequently, the other side of death remained a relative mystery because no one could describe this phenomenon with any degree of authority.

0164-0534/81/0033-0061$2.00
© 1981 Aspen Systems Corporation

62 In the last decade, a challenging approach to cardiopulmonary resuscitation, aided by modern technology in health care, has created a different perspective from which the near-death mystery may be studied. Even victims of very complex sudden death have frequently been retrieved by the rapid response and stabilization of sophisticated prehospital care and the highly effective resuscitation measures employed in emergency or special intensive care units. The present state of reversing clinical death has quickly enlarged the pool of long-term survivors, and from this group a growing number of near-death phenomena has been reported.

Although the scientific community has been slow to accept the pioneering research of investigators studying near-death events (NDEs), many postresuscitation patients have shared their perceptions of what happened to them during the clinical death phase and have thereby stimulated interest from health care professionals and lay persons alike. Literature recounting some of these early anecdotal descriptions met with added resistance because the "stories" were considered unbelievable and fantastic and were unlikely to be reproducible in a laboratory setting. However, Moody's work *Life After Life* popularized the subject and gave courage to many people who had experienced like phenomena when near death but were afraid to tell anyone.[1]

Some medical and paramedical workers admitted engaging in NDE research to refute the reports of postresuscitation victims or other clinical death survivors; instead, they proceeded to enlarge the body of NDE knowledge by collecting like reports and validating the previous accounts.[2] Finally, large circulation magazines began disseminating graphic descriptions of near-death survivors and their return to life; thus most of the Western world has been exposed in some degree to NDEs.[3]

THE RISE OF NDE RESEARCH, ASSOCIATIONS AND PUBLICATIONS

Research

During the early 1960s Osis and Haraldsson, two parapsychologists, and others engaged in an extensive and elaborate study involving over 35,000 NDE observations by soliciting reports or direct interviews from patients and care givers.[4] The survey included more than 5,000 physicians and nurses and was conducted in New York, New Jersey, Connecticut, Rhode Island and Pennsylvania. A comparison study with similar numbers of patients, physicians and nurses followed in 1972 and 1973, but Osis and Haraldsson changed the cultural variable and implemented the data collection in Northern India. Since more men than women are admitted to hospitals in India, and the mean age for Indians is lower than that for people in the United States, correctional factors were employed for comparison data analysis. The researchers' results agreed with earlier data and showed no significant differences between the reports of NDEs made by Indians and those made by U.S. respondents.[5]

Osis and Haraldsson suggested that evidence for the afterlife exists and can be divided into five major categories: (1) mediumship; (2) apparitions, especially those seen by several observers; (3) reincarnation experiences; (4) out-of-body experiences, either autoscopic or transcendental (where the "mind" is transported to other places and time); and (5) deathbed observations.[6]

Other writers and researchers have indicated a belief that life continues in some sphere after death by tallying impressive numbers of reports that describe the NDE in almost the same way as it is described by Osis and Haraldsson.[7,8] Kubler-Ross

---

The researchers' results showed no significant differences between the reports of near-death events made by Indians and those made by U.S. respondents.

---

introduced Moody's first book by announcing that over 1,500 cases of her own identified experiences of apparitions and out-of-body and deathbed revelations quite similar to those already reported in the current literature.[9]

The most comprehensive and vigorous scientific treatment of NDEs to date has been accomplished by Ring, a psychologist from the University of Connecticut. His book, *Life at Death: A Scientific Investigation of the Near Death Experience,* supports and confirms the anecdotal findings of Moody, Kubler-Ross, Oakes and others by providing these findings with overall credibility, by validating their occurrence and by drawing greater attention to them from the scientific community.[10]

Associations and publications

Amidst the growing interest in the scientific exploration of near-death phenomena, concern was expressed by a small group of researchers, writers and interested individuals to form an official organization through which data about NDEs could be shared. In 1979 the Association for the Scientific Study of Near-Death Phenomena, Inc. (now called the International Association for Near Death Studies, or IANDS) was established in Peoria, Illinois for the purpose of "collectively furthering knowledge and understanding in this long obscured realm of human experience."[11] John Audette, president of the association, and Dr. Kenneth Ring and Dr. Michael Sabom, vice presidents, invited their small contingency and all would-be members to join forces in promoting continuing scientific inquiry into phenomena associated with NDEs and the judicious clinical application of these research findings.

The organization was small, and early communication was limited to a quarterly news digest entitled *Anabiosis*. With the change and expansion of the organization, however, *Anabiosis* is changing to a biannual, research-oriented publication that will include (1) research reports; (2) theoretical or conceptual statements; (3) papers expressing a particular scientific, philosophic, religious or historical perspective on the study of NDEs and allied phenomena; (4) cross-cultural studies; (5) individual case histories with instructive unusual features; and (6) personal accounts of NDEs or related phenomena.

Four times a year, the association plans to reinstitute a newsletter-type flier, the title of which is as yet undetermined, that

64

will feature articles and materials of general interest to the members and keep them up to date on the organization's activities. Ring, editor of both publications, speculates that the newsletter will broaden in scope and become a widely circulated magazine oriented primarily toward improving and enlightening the general public about NDEs.[12]

Three other lesser-known organizations that also deal with NDEs—the International Organization for the Study of Life After Life Experiences (LUMENA), in Greenwich, Connecticut; Second Attempt at Living (SAAL), founded by Kubler-Ross in Diamond Bar, California, and the Association for Study of Life After Life, in Switzerland—are joining with similar groups already established in Spain and Scandinavia. However, the reorganized IANDS is the largest and most active group and leads the local and international collection and consolidation of scientific research and information about human consciousness and its relationship to physical death.

INFLUENCES ON NDE PERCEPTIONS

Religion and culture

Certain cogent points must be considered when attempting to understand a survivor's perceptions of the NDE. Religious and cultural practices weigh heavily on life activities, especially those integrated throughout the dying process, and may therefore be reflected in the postclinical-death report. (See "Societal/Cultural Views Regarding Death and Dying," this issue.) Krant strongly suggested that reli-

gious doctrines exert a force on people, especially the older generation, that dictates what a believer should expect after death.[13]

Other people who may not have close ties to any religious organization and are simply part of the secular society have been heard to say, "Eat, drink, and be merry, for tomorrow we die." This statement seems to imply that there is the possibility of a great void or total nothingness after the final event, so people are encouraged to "live it up" while they can. Thomas admonished his readers to carefully deliberate the likelihood of a person's annihilation or spontaneous disintegration once death is proclaimed; however, human beings generally express the need for something to believe in, a spiritual component that transcends this world and time.[14]

A brief scan of the literature of the major Western religions and their respective beliefs regarding life after death reveals that nearly all members agree that there is a supreme being, whatever name it is assigned. They probe the universe to find that person's abode (dimension) and seek to relate in some manner with that being, but they are not all convinced that a supreme god awaits them after death. Most of these Western religions incorporate ideas of heaven and hell, "out there" rewards and some kind of evaluation accompanying life's end.[15] How one lives in this world is said to dictate a person's position and place of existence in the next.

The Catholic Christian faiths go so far as to describe how one will be known on the other side of death, not by body form but by the uniqueness of personality. Even the Orthodox Jewish people, who do not practice more than five days of mourning for the deceased, are said to consider the soul immortal. They suggest that as the body deteriorates, another part of the dead person journeys to a land of deep darkness and, there, sheds individuality to become forever a part of God. Subtle fragments of these concepts have surfaced in occasional NDE reports, but none of them has done so with regularity or statistical significance.

Although a number of carefully controlled studies have specifically noted the survivor's previous religious affiliation or lack of it, no correlation has been found between the various perceptions of spiritual beings and prior religious indoctrination. Those persons describing any encounter with a supreme or angelic figure did tend to name that being with familiar religious terminology, however (e.g., God, Gabriel (angel), Jesus Christ, a Great Yellow Light). Moody suggested that some apparitions performing godlike duties might be called "Figures of Light" when no particular religious identification is made by the NDE reporter.[16]

Establishing a specific environment or position of time in which the patient suspends during clinical death has also proved unsuccessful; the greatest consensus among the NDE records supports the existence of another dimension not limited by time or material parameters. For example, the entire cardiopulmonary resuscitation procedure may take less than 60 seconds, but the patient frequently recalls a number of different events during that period.

Multiple episodes depicting various but not always chronological periods of life have been reported by persons who have experienced NDEs. Familiar statements of these individuals are: (1) "My whole life flashed before me," (2) "I remembered equally vividly those happy moments as well as the most sad times of my life . . . they were sparkling in my mind all at once but totally separate in my awareness" and (3) "I instantly knew all things over the ages, both historically and into the future." The survivor is often surprised to learn how short the actual clinical death phase lasted.

Communication

It is commonly accepted that language is a mode by which thoughts and feelings about a situation are expressed. A painting or piece of music has been suggested as an alternative way to describe phenomena "without words." Past studies of NDEs have been highly dependent on the imaginal, abstract word pictures portrayed by the survivors. Siegel stated that these "words have sensory qualities and describe such properties as sights, sounds, tastes, and smells."[17] The reported may have a comprehensive, sophisticated vocabulary or be limited and childlike when articulating the NDE.

At best, it seems to make little difference how the various components of the NDE are conceptualized, because the teller and the hearer are sending and receiving on two completely different wavelengths. The perceptions are vivid and indisputable from the patient's viewpoint, often described with a sense of near awe that the events occurred and were personal. The listener can begin to appreciate these phenomena only when the evidence is evaluated "honestly and dispassionately"

66

and free "from the tyranny of common sense."[18]

Education and formal training

Osis and Haraldsson questioned whether the less educated would report more NDE accounts than the best educated people. They found that the latter not only showed more tendency to share their stories but did so with more detail.[19]

Education may be relative to the society and the environment of the individual. Therefore, communication of what has been perceived during clinical death should show the effects of learning in a specific community—the reasoning versus the superstitions—on people who seek to understand and verbalize difficult and uncharted areas of life. Nevertheless, there is a need for other investigators to specifically analyze the respondents' level of learning along with the descriptions surrounding various components of their NDE before concluding that better educated people are more verbal about their near-fatal encounter.

Age and sex differences

Since mortality rates are greater with advancing years, common queries are, "Do adults show greater probability of experiencing NDEs at certain ages along the continuum?" and "Are children exempt from these phenomena?" A few reports of young people telling reliable witnesses and care givers of meeting dead relatives and various other apparitions suggest that some young individuals have sensed NDEs, perhaps without recognizing what these events may indicate.[20]

Retrospective accounts are cited by adults who remember an NDE in early childhood and now sense the appropriate time or place to relate it. Often, the actual recall is still so acute that the reporter does not hesitate or draw an extra breath throughout the entire statement.

Although the majority of NDE anecdotes are ascribed to adults who range in age from the late teens through the geriatric years, it has been generally accepted that members of the younger population who have been victimized by trauma probably produce the most reliable reports of their clinical-death experiences. These people tend to be healthy before their accident and without many of the variables that may alter the resuscitation response and immediate recovery period.

Physiological influences of a chemical and metabolic nature

Scientific and medical literature has clearly established that there is no one point of total organism death, but only a gradual dying process. Different organs die at various rates depending on their relative healthy or chronically diseased state. Rodin noted that a basically healthy heart can continue some type of electrical activity for 20 minutes after respiration has ceased.[21]

Current standards for best reviving a

Scientific and medical literature has clearly established that there is no one point of total organism death, but only a gradual dying process.

victim of sudden cardiac death require that cardiopulmonary resuscitation begin within four minutes of breathing and circulation cessation. From the onset of clinical death, chemical and metabolic changes may begin subtly, but the mechanisms of final organism collapse are accelerated as therapeutic interventions are unsuccessful or prolonged. Whatever illness or trauma initiated the chain of events that culminated in clinical death, the last common denominator is anoxia involving the brain.

Neurons in different locations begin degenerating with diverse celerity depending on their individual oxygen requirements. At the same time, intermediate and anaerobic metabolic pathways create less energy for the maintenance of cellular life and tip the organism away from normal physiological balance. Derangements of acid-base ratios, electrolyte ranges and body temperature add to the chemical and metabolic confusion, which may cause the mental events accompanying dying to be distorted and autolytic.

Rodin advised that the manifestations of cerebral anoxia are well known and readily reproducible in the laboratory.[22] Differences in effects are directly due to the speed with which anoxia occurs, and after a period of time, which is also variable, one lapses into unconsciousness. Rodin further noted that the first signs of hypoxia are an increased sense of peace, euphoria and power.[23] With the progression of these feelings, there is an accompanying decline in critical judgment and appropriate decision making.

If anoxia persists, delusions and hallucinations are said to occur, and eventually total unconsciousness supervenes. Likewise, certain drugs and metabolic wastes of ammonia and carbon dioxide may induce a toxic impression during the process of dying that also takes on a measure of pleasantness or conversely, total terror: "celestial spheres or the biblical bottomless pit." Rodin commented that no one has any way of predicting whether the brain in its last moments might choose to send the mind in one direction or the other.[24]

Recognizing the innumerable physiological influences that might contaminate the quality of the NDE report, Osis and Haraldsson set about identifying any clinical-death survivors who demonstrated a deviation from the normal body temperature, acid-base and electrolyte ranges and mental clarity immediately prior to their NDE.[25] The respondents were questioned and respective charts were screened to ascertain a patient's previous physiological and psychological condition, especially any mental illness, psychosis, alcoholism, uremia, brain disease, medication intoxication or mind-altering drug ingestion. The limitation of a body temperature of 103 degrees Fahrenheit was established as acceptable if the patient remained lucid.

Informally, another writer described the inclement conditions that surrounded a few patients who were on the street or in a mobile intensive care unit van and recognized that hypothermia might also affect the quality of NDE perception.[26] None of the studies surveyed paid specific attention to the immediacy of oxygen therapy during the clinical-death phase, although it is common practice to administer high concentrations of oxygen when cardiopulmonary resuscitation is initiated by prehospital emergency personnel or in-hospital

68

staff. Consequently, little is known about the exact degree of cerebral anoxia at the moment of clinical death and whether the laboratory studies coupled with educated speculations or more recent researchers can adequately present a plausible theory for the etiologies of NDEs.

Osis and Haraldsson postulated that only a small percentage of the physiological contaminants identified above were actually known to have any bearing on their patients' visions or NDE perceptions.[27] The vividness and detailed acuity of NDE reports have been questioned by several investigators and likened to certain mental states created by drugs, anesthesia of various types, hypnosis and other mind-changing modes. However, no clear and reproducible information has been collected that would support the comparison of NDE perceptions and experiences reported by other individuals who have engaged in these activities, activities of astrologic transcendence or the use of hallucinogenic compounds.

EVENTS IN THE NDE

Nearly all persons who described positive perceptions of their clinical death included some or all of the components described in the following sections though not always in the same sequence. These comments are much the same as those reported in works by Moody, Ring and others.[28-30]

A time interval without pain or peripheral feeling

In their NDE reports, patients recount an "analytical discussion" with the self about the clinical state of being alive or dead, since there is no loss of reality and the environment may remain the same. Frequently, the decision that one truly died is made because a health care giver anxiously announces, "My God, he's dead!" or "Zap him, he's straight line!" Other patients have stated that they were "relaxed," "free of pain" and "comfortable" but unaware that they had stepped from one realm to another.

The separation of mind and body

Individuals who have experienced NDEs have reported the following perceptions concerning the separation of mind and body: "A jarring, vibrating sensation went all through my body" and "the individual cells from my feet all the way to my head died, one by one; they were magnified, finely focused, brilliant, each cell flaring to a supernova and then gone.... Finally, a 'mind' floating above my body." A parting of the mind from its body may be instantaneous, with an immediate awareness of what is happening 360 degrees around the body shell. The mind may take an elevated position near the ceiling or beyond to observe what is happening to the body and which care givers are performing the various resuscitation tasks. This is known as *autoscopic observation*. Or the mind may leave the current time frame and environment to enter another age or place. This phenomenon is commonly referred to as *transcendence*.

A woman victim of a motor vehicle accident was resuscitated at the scene and again while being transported to the local emergency department. On arriving at the hospital, she frantically tried to gain the attention of a police officer investigating the case. One of the nurses attempted to comfort the patient but finally recognized that the woman wanted to communicate her concerns to the officer. Since the patient was intubated with an endotracheal tube, the nurse summoned the policeman and together they deciphered the startling message from the woman's wobbly pencil scratches on a clip board. She wrote that her husband was thrown from the car, was in a ditch about 100 feet from where she was saved, that he was dead and that we needn't hurry, but she wanted him found before daylight.[31] The policeman dispatched the message, and the rescuers found the husband exactly where the patient described him to be. Her mind had returned to the accident while she was being resuscitated by the paramedics in the mobile intensive care unit van, and she saw her dead husband's form lying in the ditch. Incidentally, she gave a precise and detailed account of the vehicles involved in the accident, including their respective damages. This was also visualized when she transcended to the accident scene.

When the mind and body separate, the mind has ultradimensional qualities unlimited by physical parameters. Patients have described their mind's ability to go through walls, follow their body on a cart to the operating room or the intensive care unit and hover outside of the window (building) to watch the resuscitation procedures from a distance. These accounts are validated by details of the facilities that correctly identify the structures, equipment, names of various items previously unfamiliar to the patients, placement of hardware and personnel within the rooms, clocks with exact time of patient entry to the area and numerous other facts that could not have been known unless the reporter of the NDE had autoscopically seen the environments in which the body was treated.

Inability to communicate to people caring for the body

Perhaps the most frustrating aspect of the entire NDE, as recounted by many survivors, is the inability to contact anyone in the medical team to express their approval and assurance that "all is being done that can be." Descriptions include how the NDE patient attempted to contact, verbalize, touch or in some way communicate that there was no pain or discomfort in the clinical-death state, that there was peace, and that the care giver should not have been upset if the resuscitation was unsuccessful. Occasionally individuals will report that they felt sadness because no one listened to the pleas of "Let me go; I am satisfied with your efforts."

One patient narrated verbatim the many conversations and associated staff behaviors during her resuscitation. At various times throughout a seven- to ten-mintue interval, the patient tried to intervene and relate the effects of various medications and procedures, along with her sentiments that she clearly understood the motives basic to each team member's actions. At one point during the clinical-death period, she described grabbing a nurse's arm when the care giver was bolusing her Lidocaine to express appreciation for administering a life-saving medicine. Later, the nurse admitted how a "strange chill" came over her when touching the patient for this intravenous injection of Lidocaine.

70

Propulsion through space or a long dark tunnel

How soon a person who is clinically dead may maneuver from one NDE phase to another is variable, not measured in earthly time and almost never self-controlled. The moves are executed rapidly, often at a propelling speed especially through the place called "a long dark tunnel," or "long dark expanse." The direction is straight ahead, rather than lateral although the body may be traveling at a distance and speed parallel to the

> *The patient may describe awakening in a beautiful meadow or heavenly place or other environment in which there is much love, warmth and brightness.*

mind. Anthony Lee portrayed a scene in which his mind was encapsulated, he experienced a "trapped feeling" and he was accelerating into the vast darkness. During that phase, Lee admitted his fright and wanted it to end or wanted to put the mind and body together for the trip.[32]

Near-death event survivors have said that movement is always of the mind, sometimes passively accompanied by its body but mostly without it. There is no one or any object close to the moving mind, although several respondents have described other forms (minds) ahead, to the side or behind the mind but unreachable and separate from what is happening to the patient's intellect. It is a singular journey. At the end of the tunnel, there is nearly always a bright light. If the NDE has not included a tunnel, but only a dark

expanse, the patient may describe awakening in a beautiful meadow, heavenly place or other environment in which there is much love, warmth and brightness.

Emergence into a place of peace, love and comfort

Propulsion through the tunnel in the NDE may include emerging into an environment of very bright, yellow, warm light. All of the vividness of this experience is indescribable, but the atmosphere has been described as a "living light." Our sunlight at its brightest is a mere shadow in comparison with this light, yet when storytellers are asked about how they could see in such brightness, they respond that " it is possible without difficulty."

The mind may be allowed to enter the bright, warm, loving area directly and converse with other members there or a deity of some kind. Or one may be held at the entrance and only allowed to see, hear and converse, perhaps about why the mind is not permitted admission at this time. The deity may indicate that "this is not the appropriate time yet" because additional earthly activities are necessary before carrying out the final residency in this place. All respondents talking about this phase, whether they were allowed to enter or not, strongly acknowledged the "living spirit" gained at this level and an overwhelming need to comply with a commitment to intensely love earthly relatives and friends upon return to the body.

Escorts to the loving, warm, bright area

If the mind is met by an escort who accompanies it to another phase, this duty is performed most often by the following entities: family members who have died and gone on before, relatives, close friends or a heavenly being or deity (various names are assigned to this being). These forms are recognized by their personalities, not their physical shapes, and they do not speak an audible language but communicate in a telepathic dimension.

The survivor of the NDE may be awestruck or feel unattached when remembering being reunited with distant relatives or little-known acquaintances and may immediately recognize that these beings use personal, intimate overtures of welcome and assistance in this realm. The various escorts may ready the patient for entrance into this environment, accompany the person from place to place, protect and perform other hospitable functions or simply welcome the traveler into the fold.

The return to the body

While the mind may wish to remain where there is love and peace, a conversation with the "spirits" or deity may alter that desire and set new directions for the return to the body and earthly reality. Rapid propulsion back through the tunnel, often in reverse rather than in a forward motion as before and without control of speed or direction, places the mind into its body. Announcement of the reunion may be made with pain, discomfort or some type of distress. It may not be comfortable to live again, but very often the new dimensions of love and caring toward one's spouse, family and friends give impetus to finish the tasks of life.

The overwhelming experience of leaving and returning to one's body is sometimes catastrophic and too much for the individual to grasp. The realization that one is

back from an experience that few other have shared places a heavy burden on the NDE survivor, and appropriate coping mechanisms are little understood by the patient and care givers alike. The patient may not show relief to be alive or may not meet the future with enthusiasm, especially when the clinical-death environment was described as pleasurable and the desire to stay in that place was very strong. Some survivors of clinical death have manifested moodiness, depression and suicidal tendencies upon returning from a magnificent NDE. Nurses must be aware that these people require a mental health assessment and probably some degree of intervention.

Negative near-death experiences

Occasionally, some victims of clinical death have related a frightening, or at best bewildering, NDE experience. The noted German actor, Curt Jurgens, described an awareness that he was in a large place or void where a shrouded, faceless figure walked toward him, lifted a hand that revealed cold, gray, icicled fingers and beckoned him to follow. Jurgens admitted that he was terror-stricken and immobilized at the spot on which he stood. As quickly as this scene was unrolled before him, it was gone. Replacing the apparition was a wall of "licking tongues of fire" that snapped out and prevented him from fleeing. Overwhelmingly afraid throughout both sequences, Jurgens told how he tried to escape but could not control any movements either by thoughts or actions. Instead, he reported feeling "alone," "trapped," "helpless" and "lost." This situation seemingly lasted "forever"; then, without indication or warning, the heinous environment was transposed into utter

72

darkness, and he lapsed into unawareness. The time of these perceptions correlated with Jurgen's cardiac arrest during open-heart surgery.[33]

Other respondents have reported glimpses of hell; bizarre creatures that attempted to devour them; entrapment within confined body parts, such as a head encapsulated within a dome and disengaged from the body; falling great distances in headfirst or backward positions; a feeling of impending doom or annihilation without an understanding of the reasons for these emotions and wandering aimlessly over desolate terrain. Most NDE survivors show trepidation while recounting their perceptions.

The memory is so vivid and real that an adult patient may beg for a family member, a nurse or anyone to constantly stay at the bedside as protection against recurrence of the terrorizing experience. Answering every patient request, from turning on bright lights 24 hours a day to dispel the darkness and administering medications to sedate the patient and tranquilize away the bad remembrances to assuring nursing support and understanding throughout the recovery period, is of little help if the NDE survivor inextricably perceives the near-fatal encounter as a personalized horror. All persons who exhibit concern about any aspect surrounding negative NDE perceptions require long-term follow-up and counseling.[34]

ENVIRONMENTS CONDUCIVE TO THE REPORTING OF NDEs

Most NDE survivors do not openly seek someone to listen to their reports because they are afraid of being labeled "crocks."[35]

The reluctance of patients to initiate discussions about near-death phenomena has been proportionate to the perceived reception to this untested information. Where the environment proved acceptable and a care giver indicated respect and belief in the patient's feelings, the story came forth like a dam breaking—creating a flood of expression, an outpouring of information.

The NDE survivor usually selects one trusted nurse, less frequently another care giver, and almost never calls for a member of the clergy to share the intimate details of near-death phenomena. Assurances are sought for confidentiality of the report, and many patients want physical signs of closed doors, quiet voices and no disclosure of information via notes or tapes as evidence that the listener respects this concern.

The NDE reporter is curious and pleased to hear that others have encountered like experiences and is generally most anxious to pass along information that may help another person later, if anonymity is preserved. Nods of relief have been frequently displayed by an NDE reporter as the listener validated a particular event or situation from notes or comments of another's NDE. There seems to be a comradery in knowing that at least a small group of people have "been there" too.

Finding a safe climate in which NDE survivors can share their experiences with family, close friends or selected agency personnel has been particularly difficult. One person stated, "Everything was black and white at home, and I never took a position on anything without a fair evaluation of the facts. My wife won't believe it's me talking." A question posed by another man was, "How will my insurance company view this report? They don't pay for psychiatric illness, you know."

An elderly woman who experienced an NDE expressed concern that her neighbors might think she was a witch with special powers and was afraid that they would try to kill her before she could hurt them. The main problem seemed to be a fear of returning home. She identified only two friends left in this world but thought they might abandon her if they knew about her NDE.

A consensus of statements by NDE survivors taken from similarly designed studies showed that patients assumed disbelief from any listener and preferred to maintain certain ties over others (i.e., keeping relationships and one's responsible position in the family were valued above any importance of telling the story to these persons). Informally, patients have stated that when they told spouses and family of the NDE and associated perceptions, they preferred to do so with a medical authority present—a nurse, mental health clinician, medical social worker or physician amenable to them. This support was viewed as providing credence and validity to the phenomena perceived by the NDE survivor and evidence that the patient was wholly lucid, appropriate and acceptable in society after experiencing the event.

NURSES' RESPONSES TO NEAR-DEATH EVENT REPORTS

Between 1975 and 1978, 30 practicing critical care and emergency nurses from a major metropolitan area that offered highly respected emergency-intensive care

services were polled for their reactions to anecdotal cases of NDE.[36] The gamut of responses included complete disbelief and skepticism, comments of "preposterous," "weird," "a scam," "hallucinations and delusions," "religious nuts" and "psychiatric blow-outs" as well as threats to expose the researcher and the study.

Some survey respondents were mildly interested but did not wish to be identified for fear that their colleagues would find

The largest group of survey returns showed the nurses to be fascinated and intensely interested in learning more about near-death event phenomena.

out and brand them as "inappropriate," and "unreliable" nurses. The largest group of survey returns showed the nurses to be fascinated and intensely interested in learning more about NDE phenomena. Approximately 50 percent of the nurses surveyed acknowledged that NDE survivors needed to report their perceptions, but they were widely divided about who should listen to the report and what that person's role is. Suggestions consisted of family members, clergy, nursing and medical personnel, the most attending care giver and a "whomever" category because the patient would ultimately select someone at random.[37]

Recording changes in any patient's clinical status is crucial to maintaining a relevant nursing care plan, but the 30 nurses disagreed about appropriate ways to utilize a patient's report of NDE. Some said that

74

they would relay the information during shift report, others acknowledged that it was important, but they were at a loss as to how it should be incorporated into nursing care.

Nurses who reviewed NDE cases in which the survivor requested anonymity and confidentiality unanimously admitted their relief of any obligation to pass along the report, yet some expressed concern that the patient may be left without an advocate and may become emotionally distressed later. Only 6 of the 30 nurses considered the NDE survivors' experiences to have an influence on all succeeding plans and care so that definite health care resources and long-range support should be offered.[38]

More recently, a small group of critical care nurses, informally surveyed using the same study design of ten anecdotal cases per nurse and noncollaborative review of each case revealed a much more open and responsive attitude toward near-death phenomena and utilization of the NDE information in planning postresuscitation care. The following questions were asked of the survey respondents:

1. What are your initial reactions to these NDE reports?
2. Comment on your perceptions of the patients' needs to share their feelings.
3. Who should be the first person to receive the patient's NDE report? Why?
4. What and how should the NDE report be recorded? For nursing care planning? For the continuing education of the health care team members? CIRCLE ONE OR MORE: (nurses, physicians, mental health workers, psychiatric staff, medical social workers, paramedics, others ___________).

The following additional questions (5–7) helped to clarify attitudes of personal involvement rather than the abstract "other nurse" references implied in questions 1–4:

5. Personalize one of the anecdotal cases to you as the nurse listener of the near-death phenomena and describe the impact on your values and attitudes about death.
6. How would you assist the NDE survivors to describe their perceptions about what they experienced during clinical death? To a respective spouse? To a respective family?
7. Would your reactions to near-death phenomena be different if one of your immediate family was the NDE reporter? How?

The questions referring to more self-examination of attitudes and feelings about NDE reports revealed unsettled feelings of the nurse respondents regarding the implication of NDE to their own death and varying degrees of anger toward the survivor who shared NDE perceptions. They generally reported being mildly angry with a family member and moderately to very perturbed with other patients. The critical care nurse group given the informal survey described themselves best able to listen, able to respond with more objectivity than any other care givers and able to provide more consistent support in dealing with issues of NDE reporting and collegial interactions but with less finesse when the patient showed signs of fear, sluggishness to "get on with living" or preoccupation with the "beautiful-loving death" perceptions.[39]

GUIDELINES FOR CARE OF PATIENTS WHO ARE POTENTIAL CANDIDATES FOR NEAR-DEATH PHENOMENA

The personnel of every unit make up different combinations of knowledge and expertise at any given time. They rotate a kaleidoscope of worthy and appropriate efforts on behalf of their patients. The following nursing care guidelines are meant only to stimulate a direction of thinking and practice for all those who venture into new dimensions of caring for NDE patients.

Since many patients have reported having NDEs during their cardiopulmonary resuscitation (CPR), the following selected guidelines have been collated to help care givers begin immediate implementation of care that is designed for potential NDE patients.

1. Station a person at the head of the patient during CPR. This care giver can provide a documentary to the patient about ongoing procedures and practice of the code team.

2. Have all code team members avoid threatening language and subliminal suggestions during and after the resuscitation. Clinically dead patients often repeat verbatim conversations and remarks made during their resuscitation. (One automobile accident victim recounted the bedside remarks accurately and imitated the German accent of one physician who responded to the code call. The patient had not previously met the physician, nor was he associated with her case or any other in the intensive care unit.)

3. Give assurance by verbal and tactile stimulation just as if the patient were awake and responsive.

4. Use comforting touch as much as possible, but be aware of how to implement this mode, especially when the patient's eyes are closed. Never touch the face and neck without notifying the patient that you plan to do so.

5. When the patient resumes consciousness, *do not abandon the patient to hardware monitoring.*

6. Begin a systematic reality orientation to time, place, person and self. Utilize patients' loved ones to orient them and the staff in recognizing subtle changes in self and personality. In a study reported by Hackett et al., nearly one-half of the patients had some type of perceptual impairment about the CPR, including confusion, disorientation and mild to severe organic brain syndrome. Many patients demonstrated difficulty in concentrating, lack of memory and slower thinking processes.[40]

7. Discuss the blackout period honestly and in matter-of-fact terms, without creating sensory overload and in "plain talk" to establish a climate for additional comments that help identify possible strange sensations and feelings about the intraresuscitation interval.

8. Do not suggest to any post-CPR patients that they really did not blackout or die if no NDE can be remembered or spontaneously recounted. Do not probe or pressure the patient for any recollections associated with the clinical-death period. Patients

may fabricate an account because they suspect that the health care team member expects some NDE report, or they may believe that they did not really die but only lapsed into unconsciousness because they did not have any of the commonly known visions.

PREPARING THE CRITICAL CARE UNIT ENVIRONMENT FOR POST-CPR PATIENTS AND FAMILIES

It is imperative that an environment that minimizes stress and the depersonalization of critical care be established for patients who have been given CPR. Nurses readily recognize that patients' surroundings strongly influence their attitudes toward illness and recovery. Unfamiliar equipment, strange facilities and staff who focus on physical problems and life support devices magnify the patient's anxieties, whereas care givers who provide frequent personal contact and comfort in conjunction with vigilant physical monitoring can do much to reduce the patient's fears that sudden catastrophe will strike again.

Although all aspects of privacy are not feasible or safely possible, post-CPR patients can be sheltered from viewing and hearing the code procedures of neighboring persons. They must be assured that nurses are available to them, that they will not be abandoned and that they are constantly monitored so that it is safe to sleep.

Patients are frequently just as anxious about the impressions that their loved ones have concerning the intensive care environment and other residents in the unit as they are about what the family believes

may be their condition. They discover very quickly that families talk together in the waiting rooms, develop support systems of sorts and exchange worries about their family member's progress or lack of it.

Post-CPR patients depend on nurses to interpret their clinical state in truthful, nondescriptive terms to their families, to provide explanations to reduce misunderstandings and to allow their families bedside access as frequently as appropriate in order to strengthen bonds of their position and love within the family structure. These mechanisms can help to establish the most facilitative climate for families to hear and accept the NDE survivor's report.

Whoever listens to the patient's description of near-death perceptions must do it attentively throughout the entire story, offer nonjudgmental comments for clarification and help associate time and events from the resuscitation with respective aspects of the NDE. Once the NDE survivor begins the account, the listener should remain impartial and attentive, no matter how incredible the report appears to be.

These actions are best provided by a nurse who is familiar with the patient's resuscitation or another member of that code team who is comfortable in answering direct questions about the CPR and related procedures. A family member

---

It is generally best for the nurse and patient to thoroughly discuss the near-death event perceptions and come to agreement on how to present them to the patient's family.

may become too emotional and thwart the reporter's story, which would thus complicate future plans and ultimately the patient's health. It is generally best for the nurse and patient to thoroughly discuss the NDE perceptions and come to agreement on how to present them to the patient's family. They can then work as a team when the perceptions are recounted to family members.

FOLLOW-THROUGH AND REFERRAL CARE FOR PATIENTS WHO HAVE EXPERIENCED NDEs

Many further comments can be made to detail care for patients after they have experienced the NDE. The following suggestions for follow-through and referral care for patients who have experienced NDEs provide minimal direction for nurses in monitoring patients' concerns that may be manifested in unhealthy coping behavior.

1. Assess the immediate postresuscitation behavior of the patient and determine the patient's levels of insomnia, restlessness and anxiety and orientation to current events and environment. Evaluate the degree of concern about the resuscitation events.
2. Utilize family accounts of a postresuscitation patient's personality changes, state of relief, depression and happiness and expressions of dependence or independence.
3. Assign each postresuscitation patient a follow-up visit by a hospital home-health care worker, especially if the patient demonstrates any behavior disturbances related to the resuscitation events.
4. Support families and postresuscitation patients who are still working through their understanding of the NDE and associated perceptions by referring them to appropriate community resources and maintaining an open line of communication through the hospital-community network.

A NEW DIMENSION FOR NURSING CARE

The era of clinical death, rapid CPR, stabilization post-CPR and long-term survivors is very young. Newer still are the reports of many "saved" patients who describe near-death experiences occurring at the moment of clinical death. Critical care team members are only beginning to know about these unusual phenomena and how they might be used in patient care plans. The nursing literature is void of background information and directions concerning the planning of post-NDE care and specific ways to evaluate if what was implemented during the resuscitation or immediately afterward altered the patient's perceptions of the NDE.

This lack of information presents a dilemma for nurses who practice in critical care areas, in which death is always imminent and holistic care is crucial. Critical care nurses must act as immediate resource persons and listen, support the patients who share out-of-the-ordinary perceptions of their resuscitations and extract data from such cases to begin building a body of knowledge about NDE.

78

The course is not easy or well marked, but nurses who practice holistic nursing care are excited about meeting this challenge. Future NDE survivors will know specific therapeutic regimens that include definite nursing care plans for dealing with these phenomena, as we now design care for postsurgical needs, infection control and mental illnesses.

REFERENCES

1. Moody, R. *Life After Life* (Atlanta: Mockingbird Books 1975).
2. Sabom, M.B. and Kreutziger, S. "Near-Death Experiences." *The Journal of the Florida Medical Association* 64:9 (1977) p. 648-650.
3. Woodward, L. "Life After Death." *Newsweek* 88: (July 12, 1976) p. 41.
4. Osis, K. and Haraldsson, E. *Deathbed Observations by Physicians and Nurses: A Cross-Cultural Survey* (New York: Parapsychology Foundation 1962).
5. Ibid. p. 45.
6. Osis, K. and Haraldsson, E. *At the Hour of Death* (New York: The Hearst Corporation, Avon Books 1977).
7. Oakes, A. "The Lazarus Syndrome: Caring for Patients Who've Returned from the Dead" in Lee, A., ed. *RN* 41:6 (1978) p. 54-57.
8. Sabom, M. and Kreutziger, S. "Physicians Evaluate the Near Death Experience." *Theta* 6:4 (1978) p. 1-6.
9. Kubler-Ross, E. "Foreword" in Moody, R. *Life After Life* (Atlanta: Mockingbird Books, 1975) p. i-iii.
10. Ring, K. *Life at Death: A Scientific Investigation of the Near-Death Experience* (New York: Coward, McCann and Geoghegan 1980).
11. The Association for the Scientific Study of Near-Death Phenomena. *Statement of Purpose* (Peoria, Ill.: The Association for the Scientific Study of Near-Death Phenomena, Inc.) p. 1.
12. Ring, K., ed. *Anabiosis* 2:3 (February, 1981) p. 1-16.
13. Krant, M. *Dying and Dignity: The Meaning and Control of a Personal Death* (Springfield, Ill.: Charles C Thomas 1974) p. 16-32.
14. Thomas, L. "Notes of a Biology-Watcher." *The New England Journal of Medicine* 292 (January 9, 1975) p. 93-95.
15. Ballou, R., ed. *The Portable World Bible* 32nd printing (Baltimore: New Viking Press 1975) p. 50.
16. Moody. *Life After Life*. p. 125-126.
17. Siegel, R. "Accounting for 'Afterlife' Experiences." *Psychology Today* 15 (January 1981) p. 65-75.
18. Rodin, E. "The Reality of Death Experiences, A Personal Perspective." *The Journal of Nervous and Mental Disease* 168:5 (1980) p. 259-260.
19. Osis and Haraldsson. *At the Hour of Death*. p. 40-45.
20. Grollman, E. *Explaining Death to Children* (Boston: Beacon Press 1967) p. 127-141, 171-195, 199-220, 223-245.
21. Rodin. "The Reality of Death Experience." p. 261.
22. Ibid. p. 261.
23. Ibid. p. 262.
24. Ibid. p. 262.
25. Osis and Haraldsson. *At the Hour of Death*.
26. Oakes, A. "Phase II of Near Death Events of Nurses." (Seattle, Wash.: Seattle Pacific University, School of Health Science, forthcoming.)
27. Osis and Haraldsson. *At the Hour of Death*. p. 55-57.
28. Moody. *Life After Life*. p. 20-70.
29. Ring. *Life at Death: A Scientific Investigation of the Near-Death Experience*.
30. Oakes. "The Lazarus Syndrome."
31. Oakes, "Phase II of Near Death Events."
32. Lee, A. "When You Know How They Feel, You'll Know What to Do" in Lee A., ed. *RN* 41:6 (1978) p. 58-60.
33. Delacour, JB. *Glimpses of the Beyond* (New York: Dell 1974) p. 200-202.
34. Oakes. "The Lazarus Syndrome." p. 55-56.
35. Moody. *Life After Life*. p. 125.
36. Oakes. "Phase II of Near Death Events."
37. Oakes. "The Lazarus Syndrome." p. 57.
38. Oakes. "Phase II of Near Death Events."
39. Ibid.
40. Hackett, R. et al. "The Coronary-Care Unit: An Appraisal of Its Psychologic Hazards." *The New England Journal of Medicine* 285 (December 19, 1968) p. 1365.

Medico-legal considerations and the quality of life

Patricia S. Davis, BS
Graduate Student
School of Nursing
Seattle Pacific University
Seattle, Washington

DEFINING DEATH

THE SOPHISTICATION of modern medicine and life-sustaining devices has brought humanity and, more specifically, those working in critical care areas, to a point of great responsibility—the determination of the criteria for death or the quality of life.[1]

Judicial history

In judicial spheres, the dilemma of defining death has surfaced in cases such as *Gray v. Sawyer*[2] and *Smith v. Smith*.[3] In both of these cases, the final conclusions of the courts were based on *Black's Law Dictionary*, which defines death as: "The cessation of life; the ceasing to exist; defined by physicians as a total stoppage of the circulation of the blood, and a cessation of the animal and vital functions consequent thereupon, such as respiration, pulsation, etc."[4]

0164-0534/81/0033-0079$2.00
© 1981 Aspen Systems Corporation

80

Smith v. Smith, however, stands out in that it was the first case in which the courts were asked to recognize brain death.[5] In this case, a husband and wife were involved in an auto accident. The husband was declared dead at the scene of the accident, but the wife was taken to the hospital unconscious, and she remained in a coma until her death 17 days later. The court petitioner argued that the couple died simultaneously because they both lost consciousness and their power of will at the same instant.[6] Although the petition was dismissed as a matter of law, the case became the basis of legislation concerning brain death in Kansas, California, Virginia, Maryland, Oregon, Georgia, New Mexico and Michigan.[7] The Michigan statute, enacted July 14, 1975, is the most succinct and thorough. It states:

8b (1) A person will be considered dead if in the announced opinion of a physician, based on ordinary standards of medical practice in the community, there is the irreversible cessation of spontaneous respiratory and circulatory functions. If artificial means of support preclude a determination that these functions have ceased, a person will be considered dead if in the announced opinion of a physician, based on ordinary standards of medical practice in the community, there is an irreversible cessation of spontaneous brain functions. Death will have occurred when the relevant functions ceased. (2) Death is to be pronounced before artificial means of supporting respiratory and circulatory functions are terminated. (3) The means of determining death in subsection (1) shall be used for all purposes in this state, including the trial of civil and criminal cases.[8]

The "relevant functions" mentioned in the Michigan law were first defined by the Ad Hoc Committee of the Harvard Medical School in 1968. The committee set forth four major criteria for the determination of brain death or irreversible coma:

1. Unreceptivity and Unresponsivity. There is a total unawareness to externally applied stimuli and inner need and complete unresponsiveness. . . . Even the most intensely painful stimuli evoke no vocal or other response.

2. No Movements of Breathing. Observations covering a period of at least one hour by physicians are adequate to satisfy the criteria of no spontaneous muscular movements or spontaneous respiration or response to stimuli such as pain, touch, sound, or light. After the patient is on a mechanical respirator, the total absence of spontaneous breathing may be established by turning off the respirator for three minutes and observing whether there is any effort on the part of the subject to breathe spontaneously.

3. No Reflexes. Irreversible coma with abolition of central nervous system activity is evidenced in part by the absence of elicitable reflexes. The pupil will be fixed and dilated and will not respond to a direct source of bright light. Ocular movement (to head turning and irrigation of the ears with ice water) and blinking are absent. There is no evidence of postural activity. Swallowing, yawning, vocalization are in abeyance. Corneal and pharyngeal reflexes are absent.

4. Flat Electroencephalogram. Of great confirmatory value is the flat or isoelectric EEG. . . . At least ten full minutes of recording are desirable, but twice that would be better. All the above tests should be repeated at least 24 hours later with no change. The validity of such data as indications of irreversible cerebral damage depends on the exclusion of two conditions: hypothermia (temperature below 90 degrees Fahrenheit, 32.2 degrees Centigrade) or central nervous system depressants, such as barbiturates.[9]

The 24 hour wait for an EEG criterion has been disputed as being unnecessary, and critics suggest that 30 minutes of no brain activity is adequate to confirm brain death.[10] These criteria imply one definition of death or life, the parameters of which are brain function. But death may be defined from several perspectives.

According to *Webster's New International Dictionary* (3rd ed.), death is "the ending of all vital functions without possibility of recovery, the end of life, the act, process, or fact of dying, the state of being no longer alive, a tasteless, joyless, dull existence, and the state of being without full possession of enjoyment of the intellectual or physical faculties."[11] This definition offers a holistic view that ranges from the end of physical growth or existence to the inability to respond, emote or be stimulated intellectually. Possibly then, according to this view, a person could be dead socially but not physically.[12]

Four approaches in defining death

Veatch, discussing the definition of death, outlines four other possible approaches:
1. the irreversible loss of flow of vital fluids;
2. the irreversible loss of the soul from the body;
3. the irreversible loss of the capacity for bodily integration; and
4. the irreversible loss of the capacity for social interaction.[13]

The irreversible loss of flow of vital fluids. This definition centers around heart and lung activity, thus a problem arises when the present use of mechanical support devices is considered. A person may be maintained on a respirator and be kept very much alive even though the person has lost lung function. The concept of death is more workable when the focus is placed on the loss of vital fluids, that is, the breath and blood. Even with mechanical support, these fluids are required for survival.

The irreversible loss of the soul from the body. This view holds that the soul forms the essential part of a person, separate from chemical or electrical forces, and it has been a key thought in historical religious tradition. The Gnostics saw salvation as being the escape of the soul from

---

The concept of death is more workable when the focus is placed on the loss of vital fluids, that is, the breath and blood.

---

the body. Christianity, in contrast, sees the body as a significant element of the person, rather than that which binds it. The loss of the soul might be considered to occur about the time the blood and breath cease circulating; the primary factor, though, is the loss of the soul. Its departure results in the cessation of fluid flow.

The irreversible loss of the capacity for bodily integration. This involves the internal environment, with its primarily unconscious homeostatic and feedback systems and the consciousness of a person, which allows the person to interact socially with other human beings.

The irreversible loss of the capacity for social interaction. This definition resulted

82

from the realization that in some instances it might be possible to lose the higher brain functions and still keep the lower brain functions necessary for such physical mechanisms as respiration. This definition raises the question of what brain capacities constitute a person's essential nature and thus determine whether that person is living.

The holders of this view would say that there are those aspects that create consciousness and allow a person to interact with others. The question is then, what level of consciousness or social interaction is significant? Do the extremely senile person and the catatonic schizophrenic individual have an adequate capacity for interaction, and if not, are they dead?

It is evident that holders of this view must avoid making such qualitative judgments. A person with a decreased ability to interact socially is not less human. Either one can interact or one cannot. Either one is alive or one is not.

Furthermore, the focus in defining death cannot rest solely on social interaction to the exclusion of the body, for the ability to relate with others operates through the body. The loss of peripheral body function cannot be the sole criterion for death, but the loss of higher functions responsible for social interaction must be contemplated in conjunction with a lack of sensation and motor response to the environment.

To complete these four definitions of death, it is necessary to determine where to look (locus) and what to look for (criteria) to decide if a person is living or dead. With the first definition, the loss of vital fluids, the loci are the lungs, respiratory tract, heart and blood vessels. The criteria are the absence of pulse or heartbeat, indicated by palpation, auscultation and an electroencephalogram, and the absence of respiration, indicated by the auscultation and visual observation (a mirror held to the nostrils).

The second definition is more complex, for it is necessary to attempt to discover the locus or seat of the soul.[14] The Bible does not specify the soul's location within a human being, only that each person possesses one and that it constitutes a personal essence. Descartes suggested that the soul resided in a small gland in the middle of the brain, and his description seems to refer to the pineal body. This creates the problem of deciding where and what to look for to see if the pineal gland has ceased to function. The Greek word *pneuma* means both "breath" and "soul or spirit," which implies that the locus of death might be in the lungs and respiratory tract. The methods of determination would then be the respiratory criteria mentioned in the first definition.

The site of bodily integration is the entire brain, which includes the cerebellum, the medulla and the brain stem. The criteria of the Ad Hoc Committee of the Harvard Medical School, mentioned previously, are those used to identify death with this concept.[15]

The locus for social interaction cannot be conclusively stated, either, but scientific evidence suggests the outer surface of the brain may be involved. With this definition, lower brain activity would have no bearing in determining death. A flat electroencephalogram would indicate loss of function in the neocortex and thus, death.[16]

THE QUALITY OF LIFE

The above discussion provides an overview of the definition of death, but with the present ability of medical science to sustain life, even when biological death seems imminent, the quality of life must also be examined. At one end of the continuum are those who would terminate life when it seems a burden or useless; at the other end are those who would preserve it at any cost.[17] McCormick attempted to present a middle position by proposing that guidelines on the quality of life be determined by examining the potential for human relationships:

Life is not a value to be preserved in and for itself. To maintain that would commit us to a form of medical vitalism that makes no human or Judeo-Christian sense. It is a value to be preserved precisely as a condition for other values, and therefore insofar as these other values remain attainable. Since these other values cluster around and are rooted in human relationships, it seems to follow that life is a value to be preserved only insofar as it contains some potentiality for human relationships. When in human judgment this potentiality is totally absent or would be, because of the condition of the individual, totally subordinated to the mere effort for survival, that life can be said to have achieved its potential.[18]

Schaeffer supports McCormick's position by reflecting on another common issue in today's society, the desire to "abort affliction":

Naturally, there is a difference between unnatural living on a machine for a long period of time and actually giving a pill or injection which would bring about death. But the whole idea of some human being's choosing exactly at what point he or she will die, or having someone in the family make that choice, is putting into existence a temptation which is too heavy for human beings to face. Whether they are family, friends or doctors of the person in question, most humans have such great weakness in the area of honest motives that they could not be trusted with such a decision .... It seems to me that what we are talking about is "Aborting Affliction."... It is a tide of temptation to put "self" first, to rate personal happiness before all else, to claim our "rights" as our basic platform and "search for fulfillment" as our purpose in life.... The problem is this: One thing swiftly leads to another. There is no stopping place when a person cuts loose from an absolute base. "Having a baby would interfere with what I want to do. Having a baby would spoil my rights. I'll abort it." But so quickly might follow: "This baby isn't perfect. Why not kill it?" And who makes the decision? And for what reasons? Abort the difficulty by killing the child? But then what is the difference when it comes to this: "I can't stand life anymore ... I'll just abort the rest of my life." And then: "How can we care for grandmother any longer? It's such a burden to us...." "... Once it becomes acceptable to decide that the quality of life is no longer worthwhile, just abort it."[19]

NURSING IMPLICATIONS

This look at the criteria for death and the quality of life is not designed to provide conclusions but to stimulate personal decision making. A nurse's philosophy ultimately recognized in daily behavior may have minimal bearing on actual patient care decisions, but a personal exploration concerning these issues can provide the nurse with a founda-

84

tion for assisting the patients, families and physicians with critical questions and for personally coping with the decisions made. Once the foundation has been laid, there are a number of practical roles that the critical care nurse can play in situations involving the "right to die" dilemma or the removal of life support systems.

A primary step in the nurse's approach to ethical issues concerning death is to have a clear understanding of state legislative and hospital policies concerning death and the termination of life support systems. These policies may involve not only criteria for death but also directives on the use of "living wills," that is, documents, signed by patients which order doctors to refrain from using life support measures that only postpone inevitable death.[20] Legislation regarding these wills has been introduced or passed in more than 40 states.[21]

A second step is to facilitate increased communication between physicians, nurses, counselors (social workers, hospice personnel, clergy) and families. On occasion, this may be especially important when the nurse recognizes that a physician is avoiding a frank conversation with a family about removing the life support system of a family member. If no family consultation has taken place and specific orders request only gradually decreasing treatment rather than palliative care, the nurse is obligated to approach the physician and other health team members for a definitive decision on the patient's behalf.

What should a nurse do if he or she suggests to the physician that he or she discuss the patient's state with the family and this suggestion is met with refusal?

These concerns need to be channeled to the appropriate nursing supervisor, the director of nursing services and the medical director of the critical care unit. The line of authority to consider regarding physician staff includes house staff, private or attending physicians and the chief of the medical staff. Each hospital has a specific chain of command, and since the issue is determining when life support equipment should be removed, it behooves the clinical nurse to assist and respect the difficult decision making process that occurs throughout all levels

---

It is very important that all members of the critical care team know the policies and boundaries concerning death within the system in which they function.

---

of critical care delivery. It is very important that all members of the critical care team know the policies and boundaries concerning death within the system in which they function.

A final step in examing issues related to the "right to die" is to participate actively in interdisciplinary committees concerned with ethical questions. A nurse who has a clear understanding of personal views and who is involved with dying patients and their families has much to offer to the policy-making process.[22]

As nursing professionals continue to face the problems of determining death and the quality of life, they require an increased understanding of their own philosophies on the issues, and they must utilize that foundation to increase communication among the health care team and patients and their families. Considerable introspection and study are expected before a nurse or other health care giver can grapple with these questions. Nurses must deal with each of these issues concerning death and the quality of life, preferably before rather than during the time that they are faced with the mental and emotional pressures of bedside decisions.

REFERENCES

1. McCormick, R.A. "To Save or Let Die." *JAMA* 229 (July 8, 1974) p. 172-176.

2. Gray v. Sawyer 247 S.W.2d 496 (Kentucky, 1952).

3. Smith v. Smith 317 S.W.2d 275 (Arkansas, 1958).

4. Beauchamp, T.L. and Perlin, S., eds. *Ethical Issues in Death and Dying* (Englewood Cliffs. N.J.: Prentice-Hall 1978) p. 14.

5. Goodman, M.R. and Aung, M.H. "Cerebral Death." *Heart and Lung* 7 (May-June 1978) p. 478.

6. Beauchamp and Perlin. *Ethical Issues in Death and Dying.* p. 14.

7. Creighton, H. "Brain Death." *Supervisor Nurse* 7(March 1976) p. 47.

8. Goodman and Aung. "Cerebral Death." p. 479.

9. Cutler, D.R., ed. *Updating Life and Death* (Boston: Beacon Press 1969) p. 56. Copyright 1968, 69, Beacon Press. Reprinted by permission.

10. "Defining Death." *Time* 105(March 10, 1975) p. 76.

11. Davis, A.J. and Aroskar, M.A., eds. *Ethical Dilemmas and Nursing Practice* (New York: Appleton-Century-Crofts 1978) p. 113.

12. Ibid.

13. Veatch, R.M. as quoted in Beauchamp and Perlin. *Ethical Issues in Death and Dying.* p. 23-33.

14. Beauchamp and Perlin. *Ethical Issues in Death and Dying.* p. 23.

15. Cutler. *Updating Life and Death.* p. 56.

16. Beauchamp and Perlin. *Ethical Issues in Death and Dying.* p. 33.

17. McCormick. "To Save or Let Die." p. 172-176.

18. Ibid. p. 172-176. Copyright 1974, American Medical Association. Used by permission.

19. Schaeffer, E. *Affliction* (Old Tappan, N.J.: Fleming H. Revell Co. 1978) p. 216-217. Copyright 1978, Edith Schaeffer. Used by permission.

20. Friedman, E. "California Hospitals Design Natural Death Act Procedures." *Hospitals J.A.H.A.* 51(November 16, 1977) p. 62.

21. Berg, D. and Isler, C. "The Right to Die Dilemma—Where Do You Fit In?" *RN(August 1977)* p. 51.

22. Davis and Aroskar. *Ethical Dilemmas and Nursing Practice.* p. 127.

Death education: a continuing process for nurses

Mary A. Seidel, RN, MS
Graduate Student
Doctoral Program in Sociology
University of Washington
Seattle, Washington

Ministry to the dying is extremely difficult if we ourselves are not quite reconciled to the truth of our own personal death. Certainly, few undertakings are more emotionally charged![1]

DEATH AND DYING have left the realm of the home and family and have become more and more the realm of the professional and the complex hospital organization. American culture today, with its emphasis on youth and life, has avoided and denied the circumstances of dying. The act of dying has lost its dignity and normalcy and has become dehumanized, mechanized and institutionalized. The growth of materialism, technology, science and individualism has made dying an individual problem and a more lonely, frightening and impersonal experience.

Unfortunately, most professionals have been socialized by this death-exorcising culture and often use their professional information and resources as a shield against unprotected encounters with death. As a result, "when physicians and

0164-0534/81/0033-0087$2.00
© 1981 Aspen Systems Corporation

88

nurses are called on to dull the sharpness of grief and to interpret death to families and survivors, they are usually unsuccessful."[2]

DEATH EDUCATION

The movement to study the social phenomenon of death and the caring processes for those who are dying evolved from a multi-disciplinary base. It has grown tremendously in the past 20 years as a result of health care practitioners' attempts to understand more about the process of dying and alleviate some of the problems and concerns that are so prevalent in working with persons who are dying.

Literature and studies on death and dying

Glaser and Strauss, Feifel, Kastenbaum, Kubler-Ross and Fulton are but a few of the individuals who have made great contributions to the knowledge and understanding of these concerns. While Feifel's book[3] opened up avenues of awareness for academicians, the time was right ten years later, in 1969, for Kubler-Ross's book[4] to open up avenues of interest and concerns for professional care givers as well as for the general public.

Many studies have been done on death and dying, and courses on these subjects have been developed for grade schools, high schools and colleges throughout the country. Journals, such as *Omega* and *Death Education*, have emerged as a forum for written communication on death-related topics. University-based centers of study have been created, and in 1976 the

Forum for Death Education and Counseling, Inc. was established to promote and upgrade the quality of death education and counseling on dying, death and bereavement.[5]

Goals for death education programs

Education about death may be defined as "a developmental process that transmits to people and society valid death-related knowledge and its implications for subsequent change in attitudes and behavior."[6] Similar to programs dealing with human sexuality, death education should be introduced in a developmental and systematic manner, for both sensitive areas have social and psychological consequences.

Leviton has identified goals that should be considered for death education. Some of the more pertinent include the following:

- Remove the taboo of death language.
- Promote appropriate interactions with the dying as human beings who are living until they are dead.
- Educate children about death so that they develop a minimum of death-related anxieties.
- Assist the individual in developing a personal eschatology by specifying the relationship between life and death.
- Assist the individual in understanding the concepts relating to a healthy death.
- Perceive the physician or counselor as a professional and human being, neither omnipotent or omniscient, who has an obligation to give competent and humane service, attention and truthful information to the dying and their families.

- Understand the dynamics of grief and reactions of differing age groups to the death of a "significant other."
- Understand and be able to interact with a suicidal person.
- Understand the role of those involved in what Kastenbaum and Aisenberg[7] call the "death system," and the assets and liabilities of that system.
- Educate consumers about the commercial death market.
- Recognize the variations involved in aspects of death both within and among cultures.
- Know the false idols and mythology existing in the growing field of thanatology, the salient heuristic questions and the great need for research.[8]

Obviously, specific goals will vary according to the target population, whether it consists of adolescents, community workers or health care professionals.

"An important conceptual point is that death education has preventive, interventive and postventive, rehabilitative capabilities."[9] It can be preventive in that it can prepare individuals and societies for subsequent events and consequences that they may experience personally and professionally. Death education can be interventive in that it can help a person who is currently facing an aspect of death and enable the person to interact more humanly and meaningfully and learn about the priorities of the dying. Finally, death education can have a postventive, rehabilitative effect when it helps a person to understand the crisis and learn from that experience.[10]

From a societal standpoint, it appears that death education is not only beneficial but has become a necessary aspect of socialization. Given the current attitudes about death in our country and mechanisms of the health care system, "the time is ripe for death education to assume a proper role in our cultural upbringing as a preparation for living."[11]

DEATH EDUCATION FOR NURSES

The nurse is the health care professional who has the highest degree of contact with dying persons and their families. The

---

The nurse is the health care professional who has the highest degree of contact with dying persons and their families.

---

majority of nurses work in hospitals, and it is in these hospitals that most people die.

Nurses are expected to react differently to death and dying than other individuals do. They are expected to be capable of providing reassuring and humane care for the critically and chronically ill.[12] With this expectation, nurses face a dilemma. Young professionals are in no way exempt from the conditioning of their own past experiences in a culture that is uneasy about the events of death and dying.[13] They are asked not only to provide physical care for dying patients but also to provide for their patients' and families' understanding, comfort and support in circumstances that are unfamiliar to them and contrary to their early socialization. Conflicts frequently surface when nurses begin to confront this uncomfortable dilemma.[14]

Improving the care for the dying and reducing the conflict that surrounds this care are challenges for nursing education. Of the many nurses who have contributed to the field of death education and care of the dying, a few can be considered "pioneers." In 1959 Saunders wrote a series of articles about dying people, euthanasia, the care of the dying and nursing approaches to these and related problems.[15-20] Quint, in her writings about nurses and dying patients, drew attention to the importance of nurses considering dying patients as distinct from other patients.[21] Her work and the writings of Folta have influenced the approach to caring for dying persons and the education of nurses regarding the process of dying.[22]

Planning educational programs for nurses

Several factors can influence the planning of death education programs for nurses. First, learning about death and dying should be considered *a continuous process* that cannot be achieved after one course, at one workshop or in writing one paper. At different times in their professional careers, nurses may have various experiences with the dying and frequently express different concerns about caring for these dying persons. These experiences vary with the settings in which nurses work, for the nature of and contact with death is vastly different in community health, hospice care and critical care units.

A second factor to be considered in planning for the continuing educational needs of nurses caring for dying persons and their families is the role conflict that

nurses may encounter as they bridge their personal and professional worlds. There is a real need to consider the personal characteristics of individual nurses, such as educational level, age, religious affiliation and ethnic origin,[23-25] as these influence nurses' perceptions of death and dying. These personal characteristics contribute to how individuals "see their world" and, subsequently, their professional role. At times, a nurse's personal beliefs or experiences may enhance or hinder professional responsibilities; it is therefore important to understand and appreciate the relationship between these two aspects of a nurse's life.

There are occasions when situations in personal lives override and interfere with relations with patients and colleagues (such as illness or death in the family). By achnowledging these influences, nurses can better determine ways to deal with them. Ignoring them or discounting them as "unprofessional," as was the method of the past, does not eliminate these influences, for they frequently emerge in more diffuse and subtle ways in interactions with patients and other staff.

When considering death education for nurses, a difficult area to deal with emotionally, it is important to address personal conflicts with professional responsibilities and offer opportunities for nurses to express these concerns and work out reasonable solutions. For example, if a nurse has been having problems in his or her family, the nurse may have less patience to work with a patient who has been in a great deal of pain and is very irritable. The resolution of this problem may be that this particular nurse work with several ambulatory, less demanding patients for a few days until pressures have been alleviated at home. At this point, the nurse might well be ready to resume the care of the more difficult patient and can thus offer a relief for his or her colleague, who has been carrying a heavy patient load.

The need for education about death and dying continues throughout a nurse's career, but the specific types of educational experiences needed differ with each stage of that career and in relation to the personal characteristics and experience of each individual.

Stages in professional development

Whether or not careers in nursing are well planned and continuous or spontaneous and interrupted, nurses tend to pass through various stages in their professional development. These stages provide a framework for looking at the continuing changes that nurses may encounter as they assume various positions in nursing service and education.

The following four suggested stages of nursing have not been articulated in the literature, but have been derived from observations and clinical experience:

1. the professional nursing student;
2. the professional nurse in beginning practice;
3. the experienced professional nurse involved in direct patient care; and
4. the advanced professional nurse involved in indirect patient care.

Each of these stages in the nursing professional's career determines the varying needs of nurses in that position and the

subsequent nature of the educational experiences that might be planned for them.

The professional nursing student

In a 1978 study of 205 schools of nursing in the United States (bachelor's degree, associate degree and diploma programs) only 5 percent reported that they offered a required course on death and dying; 39.5 percent indicated that an elective course on this subject was available for their students.[26] Some schools chose to integrate concepts of death and dying into their curriculum, but often this integration was limited to an occasional lecture in one or two courses.

As a result of the limited availability of death education for nursing students, these students may have little knowledge about the process of dying and the needs of the dying patient. It may also be common for nursing students to complete their basic education without having personally witnessed a death or without having had contact with terminally ill patients and their families. Moreover, it appears that there is a first generation of young people in the United States who have grown to adulthood without ever having experienced a death in their immediate families.[27] Therefore, although death and the care of the terminally ill are almost daily occurrences in most U.S. hospitals, it appears that many contemporary nursing students have limited knowledge about and little or no direct exposure to these phenomena.

Nursing educational programs must provide students with beginning skills and an understanding of the dying process and

92

an appreciation for the conflicts this process arouses in society at large and in the health care institution specifically. These skills are basic in the preparation for the generalist role of the RN.

All nursing students should have the opportunity to work with a dying patient and his or her family at least once during the nursing program so that they can receive the necessary support, supervision and guidance from clinical faculty. Too often the recent graduate must face this first professional encounter with death alone and without support and supervi-

---

Faculty must recognize that skills in working with dying patients are essential regardless of a nurse's clinical specialization or work setting.

---

sion. This situation results from an inadequacy in basic nursing education and needs to be eliminated or at least reduced.

Several steps are necessary in preparing nursing students for work with the dying. First and foremost, it is essential that faculty acknowledge the importance of the nursing role in caring for the dying and their families. Faculty must recognize that skills in working with dying patients are essential regardless of a nurse's clinical specialization or work setting. The teaching of the necessary skills and knowledge can be incorporated into the curriculum in a specific course or can be integrated into the core courses.

For faculty members to incorporate death education into the nursing program, they must be comfortable with the subject matter themselves and competent to work with students in this area. Often, meaningful experiences are overlooked and important learnings ignored because of a lack of interest, abilities or understanding on the part of the clinical faculty.

If death education is not part of the curriculum of a nursing school, various solutions can be explored. First, faculty who are interested and prepared can volunteer to offer these experiences to their students. Second, experts can offer faculty workshops and clinical experiences that would prepare interested but ill-equipped faculty in this area of care. Third, faculty can be encouraged to use nurse clinicians and staff in various clinical settings to work with and supervise students in caring for the dying patient.

It should be remembered that many faculty were originally socialized in nursing 20 to 30 years ago, when death education included postmortem care and directions to the pathology lab or the mortuary. Content on death and dying in both bachelor's and master's degree programs remains limited. Even when faculty continued their education, they may not have had the opportunity to learn more about care of the dying person or to deal with the reactions and feelings toward death that they had when they were students and young staff nurses.

Selection of clinical settings that provide opportunities for students to work with dying persons can be problematic. Intensive care units, in which patients are often acutely ill and near death, may not be the best settings. These units are small and are frequently crowded with staff and equipment, which makes supervision difficult. The intensity of the work in such units and the emergency nature of impending death adds to the anxiety of the student.

On the other hand, hospice centers and special units in hospitals, such as oncology and pediatric hematology, may provide rich environments for students to work with dying persons. In these settings death is expected and considered a necessary outcome and natural process. In addition, the staff, specialists working with the dying, can serve as role models in giving care to these individuals. A supportive, nurturing environment for patients will be the least stressful setting for beginning students to learn about death and their role in caring for the dying and their families.

Both faculty and clinical staff need to remember that nursing students are just beginning to gain a sense of their identity, both personally and professionally, since they are usually in late adolescence or early adulthood (though this predominant age pattern has changed considerably in the past decade). The students need to focus on mastering basic physical assessment tasks, comfort measures and the administration of medications and treatments, as well as basic communication skills.

It is important to maintain reasonable expectations for beginning-level nursing students and offer them the opportunity to work with other professional staff or faculty in caring for dying patients and their families. When offering a nursing student the opportunity to work with dying patients, faculty should make themselves available to the student in the clinical setting, at school or by home telephone

so that the student will have emotional support. Through this communication, students can acknowledge and begin to deal with their feelings about patients and their families and with their own sense of competency.

If a faculty member is going to work with an individual student who is caring for a dying patient, the faculty member must also make arrangements for some staff members to supervise the other students in the clinical group. This type of arrangement requires that the faculty member and the agency staff have a positive working relationship that involves an open communication system and respect for each other's role and competence. Clinical seminars and nursing rounds can also be planned as useful opportunities for students, faculty and staff to share their feelings about working with particular patients on the unit who are dying and to plan and evaluate their care.

The professional nurse in beginning practice

The transition from a nursing student one day to a graduate nurse the next is often very threatening. The orientation program in a health care agency can play a critical role in reducing the tensions and fears of this role transition. As noted before, nurses often come to their first position with little or no experience in working with dying patients. The orientation program would be an ideal time to offer this experience to the new graduate.

The orientation program could include the following:

- theory classes about the process of dying;

94

- review of the code cart;
- practice with equipment, medications and routine emergency treatments (tasks that may be frightening to new graduates); and
- an opportunity to work with another staff nurse, in-service instructor or clinical specialist in caring for several dying patients and their families.

Staff conferences and patient presentations would also be helpful during this first year of nursing practice. Clinical supervisors, head nurses and team leaders can make themselves available to new graduates in helping them develop the physical and psychosocial skills that are so necessary in working with the dying. One factor that will influence these experiences will be the real and expected occurrence of death on a particular unit. Deaths may be frequent and expected or may occur only once in a while in an emergency situation. Experiences in the orientation program could explore these differences with each new staff member.

It is also important to remember that nurses in this stage of professional development may also be older nurses who are returning to the field or changing specialties after a long absence. These nurses should be given beginning support when caring for the dying patient, similar to that given to the new professional nurse, until the returning graduate feels ready to assume increasing responsibility. It is also important to realize that the life experience of these "more mature" nurses may be rich and may allow them to better understand and communicate with the dying patient, even though their initial training provided little preparation for working with the dying.

The experienced professional nurse involved in direct patient care

Once the professional nurse has developed basic technical and psychosocial skills, he or she may decide to move to another unit or agency or may advance to another, more responsible role, such as team leader, clinical specialist or clinical instructor. Such advancement usually requires increased competence in a particular area, with specialization in theory and practice. This stage may involve a return to school for further formal education.

More experienced nurses have expanded their personal and professional knowledge and skills and may have been confronted with other, perhaps conflicting, ideas, values and philosophies about the care of dying patients and their families. At this time, these nurses may be ready to expand their narrower focus on the patient and family to include other professionals on the health care team and the institutional practices and policies that may be influencing the interactions.

More secure in their own knowledge and skills, these nurses can now deal with death-related situations more effectively and can allow patients and their families more control over their own care. Issues about personal competence are less significant, whereas methods for managing a situation in the most appropriate manner emerge as important concerns.

Nurses in this phase of their career may well benefit from more in-depth inservice programs, workshops and continuing education options. University courses at the graduate level should be available for students to study death as a social phenomenon and its implications for care.

At this stage, nurses may see the need for change and may develop specific programs for improved care or write about some aspect of their clinical practice for publication.

In the clinical setting, staff conferences remain a valuable experience. When death is a common occurrence on a particular unit, counselors might be made available to staff for weekly seminars or on an individual basis to discuss feelings and concerns about particular patients and their care.

In some hospitals, nurses have been encouraged to attend wakes and or funerals of deceased patients as a mechanism for providing closure to professionals and family members regarding the loss of the family member and patient. Often families visit the unit on "anniversary" dates, which also provides opportunities for both family and staff to share their feelings and concerns. These practices are not only beneficial for experienced nurses in clinical practice but may help nurses at all stages in their professional careers.

Another valuable approach in death education for nurses who provide direct patient care is to encourage faculty in nearby schools of nursing to act as educational resource persons for a particular unit. This is another way to help bridge the gap between nursing education and practice, with a shared goal for improved patient care.

The advanced professional nurse involved in indirect patient care

The last stage of the professional nursing career includes those nurses who are in leadership positions that do not involve

Most professional nurses involved in indirect patient care function independently and may therefore need support groups in which they can discuss mutual concerns about the care of dying patients.

direct patient care, such as administration, education, consultation and research. Although these nurses are not directly involved in caring for dying patients and their families, they are often responsible for changing the system of care. These changes can occur through curriculum revision, academic writing, policy or legislative changes or the development and implementation of research studies that relate to the care of the dying patient.

Most professional nurses involved in indirect patient care function independently and may therefore need support groups in which they can discuss mutual concerns about the care of dying patients. The notion of collegiality is important at this level of a nurse's career. A support group could involve regional planning and coordination for the following: (1) developing educational programs, (2) providing consultation, (3) offering workshops and courses to other professional groups and auxilliary workers and (4) encouraging the collaboration of several agencies in clinical research.

DEATH EDUCATION AND IMPLICATIONS FOR NURSING

That certain types of educational experiences are discussed under a particular stage of professional nursing development

96 in this article does not preclude the possibility that nurses at other levels of professional development can benefit from these experiences. This exchange would further increase the amount of understanding and communication between various roles in nursing—the staff nurse, the dean, the researcher and the student.

The ongoing nature of learning in the nursing field as nurses develop both personally and professionally reinforces the continuing process of death education. Various programs and learning experiences must be available to professional nurses who are dealing with the care of dying patients and their families. The various opportunities reflect needs that arise from the nurse's role or position in the organization, the nurse's level of expertise, the setting in which practice occurs and the individual characteristics and personal experiences of the professional. These programs are a *joint* responsibility of nursing education institutions and service agencies in their *mutual goal* of improving the quality of care given to dying persons and their families.

In one of Thoreau's last essays, "Autumnal Tints," he describes how leaves decay and bring forth new life: "They teach us how to die. One wonders if the time will ever come when men, with their boasted faith in immortality, will lie down as gracefully and as ripe . . . ." Perhaps educational programs for nurses who work with the dying can facilitate this process.

REFERENCES

1. Feifel, H. "Death and Dying in Modern America," *Death Education* 1:1 (1977) p. 12.
2. Ibid. p. 5-14.
3. Feifel, H., ed. *The Meaning of Death* (New York: McGraw-Hill 1959).
4. Kubler-Ross, E. *On Death and Dying* (New York: McMillan 1969).
5. Pine, V.R. "A Socio-Historical Portrait of Death Education." *Death Education* 1:1 (1977) p. 57-84.
6. Leviton, D. "The Scope of Death Education." *Death Education* 1:1 (Spring 1977) p. 44.
7. Kastenbaum, R. and Aisenberg, R. *The Psychology of Death* (New York: Springer 1972) as quoted in Leviton. "The Scope of Death Education." p. 44.
8. Leviton. "The Scope of Death Education." p. 44-45.
9. Ibid. p. 47.
10. Ibid. p. 45-47.
11. Feifel. "Death and Dying in Modern America." p. 11.
12. Thrush, J.C. and Paulus, G.S. "The Availability of Education on Death and Dying: A Survey of U.S. Nursing Schools." *Death Education* 3:2 (1979) p. 131-142.
13. Wise, D. "Learning About Dying." *Nursing Outlook* 22:1 (1974) p. 42-44.
14. Martin, L. and Collier, P. "Attitudes Toward Death: Survey of Nursing Students." *Journal of Nursing Education* 14:1 (1975) p. 28-35.
15. Saunders, C. "Part I: Care of the Dying: the Problem of Euthanasia." *Nursing Times* 55 (October 9, 1959) p. 960-961.
16. Saunders. "Part II: Should a Patient Know?" *Nursing Times* 55 (October 16, 1959) p. 994-995.
17. Saunders. "Part III: Control of Pain in Terminal Cancer." *Nursing Times* 55 (October 23, 1959) p. 1031-1032.
18. Saunders. "Part IV: Mental Distress in the Dying." *Nursing Times* 55 (October 30, 1959) p. 1067-1068.
19. Saunders. "Part V: The Nursing of Patients Dying of Cancer." *Nursing Times* 55 (November 6, 1959) p. 1091-1092.
20. Saunders. Part VI: When a Patient is Dying." *Nursing Times* 55 (November 13, 1959) p. 1129-1130.
21. Quint, J.C. "Awareness of Death and the Nurses' Composure." *Nursing Research* 15:1 (1966) p. 49-55.
22. Folta, J. "The Perception of Death." *Nursing Research* 14:3 (1965) p. 232-235.
23. Gaston, S.K. "Death and Midlife Crisis." *Journal of Psychiatric Nursing and Mental Health Services* 18 (January 1980) p. 31-35.
24. Kalish, R.A. and Reynolds, D.K. "The Role of Age

in Death Attitudes." *Death Education* 1:2 (1977) p. 205-230.

25. Kalish, R. and Reynolds, D. *Death and Ethnicity: A Psycholcultural Study* (Los Angeles: University of Southern California Press 1976).

26. Thrush and Paulus. "The Availability of Education on Death and Dying: A Survey of U.S. Nursing Schools." p. 131-142.

27. Fulton, R. "The Sociology of Death." *Death Education* 1:1 (1977) p. 15-25.

Book reviews

Catherine Hogan, RN, MSN
Assistant Professor of Nursing
La Salle College
Philadelphia, Pennsylvania

Lois W. Lowry
Doctoral Candidate
University of Pennsylvania
Philadelphia, Pennsylvania

Marylou K. McHugh, RN, MSN
Counselor, Department of Nursing
La Salle College
Philadelphia, Pennsylvania

Mary Timpe, RN, MN
Thomas Jefferson University
Philadelphia, Pennsylvania

New Meanings of Death edited by Herman Feifel. New York: McGraw-Hill Co. 1977. *355 pages, $7.95.*

This thought-provoking text explores death in contemporary America, death and development throughout the life span, clinical management, survivors and responses to death. Each chapter is significant, and the entire text is unique. This is because this compilation of works reflects many diverse professional attitudes and beliefs on death and dying.

The tone of the text is set in the introduction. Herman Feifel discusses the ramifications of technological change on people's perceptions of death and the process of dying. He points out that the public's perspective has been affected by advances in medicine and by television's portrayal of death in news coverage of wars and violent crime. The concept of death is often accepted as an impersonal statistic. Technology has also changed the process and locale of dying and has

1064-0534/81/0033-0099$2.00
© 1981 Aspen Systems Corporation

100

alienated many from traditional moorings, weakening family and community supports.

Dr. Avery Weisman points out that consumer activism has caused the challenging of established ways, products and ideas regarding death and dying. Other authors discuss issues reflecting this distrust of the public including the concepts of voluntary euthanasia, living wills and funerary practices. The questioning of the professional competence of the care giver and of health care institutions has given rise to the need for informed consent.

The chapter, "Death and the Physician," by Dr. Laurens White looks at the medical profession, pointing out the shortcomings of physicians who see their role as curing, not caring. White discusses semantics and recommends that physicians avoid the loose use of the word "terminal" as it has an emotional impact for both the individual and the physician. Frustration and anger affecting the physician–patient relationship emerge when death of another affects the context in which one views his or her own death. For the care giver the reality of dying evokes feelings of failure and helplessness. White advocates open discussion of diagnosis with patients and family together to decrease potential communication barriers. He explores denial through presentation of a clinical situation illustrating that individuals may know they are dying, but not believe it as they have chosen not to deal with it. This emotional resistance to the illness is an individual's choice, but without knowledge the client is deprived of this resistance option.

In this text all the authors speak frankly on death and dying from their varied professional perspectives reflecting the open appraisal of attitudes prevalent in medicine today. This book is recommended for all who care for dying people and for all people who care.

—Catherine Hogan

The Hour Of Our Death by Philippe Aries. New York: Knopf 1981. *614 pages, $20.00.*

The *Hour of our Death* is a search into the attitudes toward death manifest in Western Christian culture. The author hypothesizes that as humans have become more focused on their individuality, death has become a less important phenomenon. He has searched cemeteries, church records, wills, literature, theological and sociological documents in European countries, and has studied modern funerary customs to test this hypothesis.

The scope of this research is 1,000 years—from the 10th to the 20th centuries. The rationale for this extended search is to detect subtle changes in attitudes from century to century.

The author has included both intuitive and subjective methods among his research tools, interpreting beyond the intent of the writers and artists to the unconscious expression of the sensibility of the age.

The book is divided into five parts, each of which is concerned with four recurrent themes: the awareness of the individual, the defense of society against untamed nature, belief in an afterlife and belief in the existence of evil. Each of the five book sections is concerned with a different period in history and traces the attitude, celebration and symbolization of death during each period.

In the decade of the early Christian era, death was too familiar to be frightening. It was accepted and announced, each life subordinate to the community that celebrated the death rituals and then resumed its functions. In the 11th century the elite and educated advocated the importance of self. With death of the self, there developed a growing fear of the afterlife and belief in the concept of a last judgment. Christian beliefs dictated the behaviors and rituals surrounding death in this era.

During the Renaissance, society began to view death as violent and savage. The family unit surpassed the community in importance. Passionate attachments and deep grieving surrounded the death of the lost loved one. Physicians replaced clergy in expressing ideas about death and the care of the dead body. The desire for knowledge of anatomy encouraged grave robbing and embalming practices.

In the 20th century death has become a private affair, the dying are removed to an impersonal hospital where even they are protected from the knowledge of their impending death.

Aries, a Frenchman, intending this work for an American audience whose preoccupation with death has become increasingly evident in the past decade, has accumulated information from a myriad of sources. However, it is difficult to identify the themes from era to era. This may be due to the difficulties inherent in translation. The data do support his hypothesis that as humans have become more self-centered, death has become less important. And the author acknowledges the efforts of some in our modern world who wish to return to the acceptance of death as a part of life, and to remove the fears, terror and violence surrounding it.

However, death is a fact of life and theologians, thanatologists and health care professionals must still deal with it. The information presented here provides them with an understanding of the meanings and rituals surrounding death through the ages.

—Lois W. Lowry

Heartsounds by Martha Weinman Lear. New York: Pocket Books, 1981. *501 pages, $3.50.* New York: Simon and Schuster 1979. *413 pages, $12.95.*

Heartsounds is the story of Harold Lear, urologist and sexual therapist—of his fight for life against profound cardiac disease and against the dehumanizing process known as the miracle of modern medicine. Although steeped in medical tradition, both Lear and his wife were constantly surprised and angered by a system they understood but were unable to penetrate when Lear became a patient.

From the onset of his illness Lear encountered difficulty choosing a cardiologist. Being new to the area and not part of a close professional family, he had to select a physician in much the same way as any lay person. Many physicians were suggested, but ultimately Lear chose a cardiologist recommended by a nurse with whom Mrs. Lear was acquainted.

At the hospital, no one assessed Lear

102

well enough to find the answers he wanted. He felt that the physicians heard what they wanted to hear and responded accordingly, not really listening to the patient. The cumulative effects of the many drugs he was taking were not checked, and the interactions of these drugs were not explained. The physicians' attitudes seemed to be that Lear's cardiac arrest was his own fault. Lear began to wonder how the average patient survived medical treatment.

In contrast to the physicians' treatment, nursing care seemed so positive. Nurses became more important to Lear than the physicians. They were honest, seemed to understand how he felt about what was happening to him and shared these insights with his wife. She in turn felt less anxious. Because he did not know the scope of nurses' responsibilities, he found them compassionate and blameless. He was unaware that they could have assessed his pain, given him aspirin rather than meperidine and educated him concerning his drug regimen. Would he have had less difficulty with his medical management if he had had a primary nurse, a clinical specialist, as advocate?

This book is powerful, objectively dealing with inadequacies in the medical system. The rage felt by the Lears was valid; yet the tone of the book is one of passive acceptance with few outbursts of aggression. The Lears are sensitive people who accepted the power of the system.

Nurses will find much that is thought provoking and enlightening as they read this book.

—Marylou K. McHugh

Learning to Say Good-by by Eda LeShan, illustrated by Paul Giovanopoulous. New York: Avon Books 1978. *124 pages, $2.95.*

Learning to say Good-by is designed to fill a void in American society. Few people have much experience with death, often reaching adulthood without losing someone close to them. Since adults may not know how to handle death, they may find it difficult to help a child through the same experience.

This book is directed to the school-aged child, from the age of eight years on, who has lost a parent. The author describes the feelings surrounding the death of a parent, beginning with shock and denial and continuing on through the period of grieving, to the stages involved in recovery. She points out the way children may react to a death (such as feeling anger and guilt) and discusses how adults may helpfully respond to the child. Not all adult advice is positive, although it is probably well intentioned.

The material in this book is presented in a factual manner with the use of numerous case studies to personalize the experience of death for the young reader. One study describes the situation of two sisters, one 13 and the other 8 years of age. The author tells how the older girl's friends supported her because they were mature enough to understand some of her feelings while the younger child's peers could not cope with the idea of the loss and avoided her. How the younger child's pain is resolved and how, in time, she found new friends who understood her is discussed.

This book will be useful in helping a

child reach some understanding of his or her feelings about the death of a parent. It can be quite helpful immediately after the death in preparing the child for the emotions he or she may experience. However, since not all children are equipped to confront their feelings immediately, the book can be made available a little later for them to read and think about at their own pace.

This book is complete in itself, and a similar book could be written to help siblings accept the death of a brother or sister. The limitation of the book is that it concentrates on middle-class children from organized stable families, and parental death occurs in all economic groups. *Learning to Say Good-by* can be used as a basis for discussion by nurses who work with groups of children or with the dying. The best use of the book is as a common ground for those in a family who have shared the loss of a member as sharing the grief helps many people work through their pain.

—Mary Timpe

Notices

All material to be considered for publication in Notices should be addressed to: Editor, Notices, TCN, Aspen Systems Corporation, 1600 Research Boulevard, Rockville, MD 20850.

ADDICTIVE BEHAVIOR TREATMENT CONFERENCE

The Department of Psychology of the University of New Mexico is sponsoring the Grand Canyon International Conference on Treatment of Addictive Behaviors on November 17-21, 1981. Alcoholism, drug abuse, smoking and obesity will be the areas covered. The program content will be of primary interest to psychologists, physicians, nurses, social workers and counselors involved in those areas. Invited speakers will include internationally known figures in the field. For further information on this conference contact: William R. Miller, PhD, Program Chair, Grand Canyon International Conference, Department of Psychology, The University of New Mexico, Albuquerque, NM 87131.

APON CONFERENCE

The Association of Pediatric Oncology Nurses is sponsoring a workshop on Current Issues in Pediatric Oncology: Legal and Ethical Aspects of Treatment for the Child or Adolescent with Cancer. The meeting will be held on October 29 and 30, 1981, at the Hyatt on Union Square in San Francisco, California.

Tuition is $75.00 per member, $100.00 per nonmember and $65.00 per student. Application has been made for ten continuing education contact hours. For further information contact: Margaret Stewart, RN, MA, National Program Chairman, Association of Pediatric Oncology Nurses (APON), c/o Illinois Cancer Council, 36 South Wabash Avenue—Suite 700, Chicago, IL 60603.

PEDIATRIC CARE WORKSHOPS

The Children's Hospital of Philadelphia is sponsoring several pediatric care workshops for the academic year 1981-1982. The first meeting is October 1 and 2, 1981, on the subject of Neonatal Ophthalmology. The tuition is $150.00 for 12 hours of credit.

For a list of future sessions, their dates and tuition fees, contact: P.S. Pasquariello, Jr., MD, Director, CME, The Children's Hospital of Philadelphia, 34th & Civic Center Blvd., Philadelphia, PA 19104, (215) 596-9548.

OPERATING ROOM CRISES WORKSHOP

The School of Nursing of the University of Southern Mississippi is sponsoring a workshop entitled "Nursing Care of Patient who Experiences Crises in the Operating Room." This course is designed to expand the nurse's knowledge base when caring for patients who experience complications in the operating room. The focus is on restoration, stabilization or regulation of integrated functioning.

The workshop will be held November 14, 1981 at the University of Southern Mississippi School of Nursing in Jackson, Mississippi. The program is accredited by the Central Regional Accrediting Committee of the American Nurses' Association for 5 contact hours. The fee is $26.

For further information contact: Mrs. Jesse Lee Stevens, Coordinator of Workshops and Conferences, Continuing Education Program, University of Southern Mississippi, Southern Station, Box 5104, Hattiesburg, MS 39401.